PHOTOGUIDE TO DRUG ADMINISTRATION

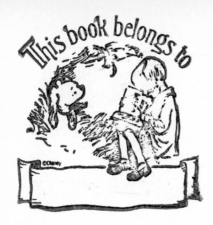

This book belongs to

PHOTOGUIDE TO DRUG ADMINISTRATION

SPRINGHOUSE CORPORATION
Springhouse, Pennsylvania

Staff

Executive Director, Editorial
Stanley Loeb

Editorial Director
Helen Klusek Hamilton

Clinical Director
Barbara McVan, RN

Art Director
John Hubbard

Clinical Editors
Patricia Holmes, RN, BSN, Paulette Dorney, RN, MSN, CCRN

Copy Editor
Mary Hohenhaus Hardy

Drug Information Editor
George J. Blake, RPh, MS

Editorial Assistant
Beverly Lane

Designers
Stephanie Peters (associate art director), Jacalyn Facciolo, Donna Giannola, Susan Hopkins Rodzewich

Photographer
John Gallagher

Illustrators
Jean Gardner, Bob Jackson, Judy Newhouse, Bob Newman, Larry Ward

Art Production
Robert Perry (manager), Anna Brindisi, Donald Knauss, Tom Robbins, Robert Wieder

Manufacturing
Deborah Meiris (manager), T.A. Landis, Jennifer Suter

Production Coordination
Colleen M. Hayman

Indexer
Barbara Hodgson

PGDA-010792

LIBRARY OF CONGRESS CATALOGING-IN-PUBLICATION DATA
Photoguide to drug administration/contributors and reviewers.
  Leslie Ann Clark ... [et al.].
    p. cm.
  Includes bibliographical references and index.
  1. Drugs–Administration–Handbooks, manuals, etc. 2. Nursing–Handbooks, manuals, etc. I. Clark, Leslie Ann. II. Springhouse Corporation.
III. Title: Photoguide to drug administration.
  [DNLM: 1. Drug Administration Routes–atlases. 2. Drug Administration Routes–nurses' instruction. 3. Drugs–administration & dosage–atlases. 4. Drugs–administration & dosage–nurses' instruction. QV 17 P575]
RM147.P53 1992
615.5'8–dc20
DNLM/DLC   91-4881
ISBN 0-87434-365-8   CIP

Contents

Contributors and consultants

Leslie Ann Clark, RN, MSN
Clinical Nurse Specialist, Pain Management Service
Department of Anesthesiology
University of California
San Diego

Doris A. Millam, RN, CRNI, MS
I.V. Therapy Clinician
Holy Family Hospital
Des Plaines, Ill.

Alice S. Poyss, RN, PhD
Assistant Professor
College of Nursing
Villanova (Pa.) University

Donna Starsiak, RN,C, MSN
Assistant Professor of Nursing
Niehoff School of Nursing
Loyola University of Chicago

Acknowledgments

The editors gratefully acknowledge the kind cooperation of the following people and companies during preparation of this volume.

Abbott Laboratories
Hospital Products Division
Abbott Park, Ill.

Ambler Pharmacy
John McVan, Pharmacist
Ambler, Pa.

Applied Biotech Products, Inc.
Lafayette, La.

Arrow International, Inc.
Reading, Pa.

Bard Interventional Products
C.R. Bard, Inc.
Billerica, Mass.

Baxter Pharmacy Division
Baxter Healthcare Corporation
Deerfield, Ill.

Bird Products Corporation
Palm Springs, Calif.

Catheter Technology Corporation
Bloomington, Ind.

Cook Critical Care
Barbara Stewart, Technical
  Marketing Assistant
Bloomington, Ind.

Data Chem, Inc.
Indianapolis, Ind.

Davol, Inc.
Subsidiary of C.R. Bard, Inc.
Cranston, R.I.

Fisions Corporation
Rochester, N.Y.

Geigy Pharmaceuticals
Division of CIBA-GEIGY
  Corporation
Ardsley, N.Y.

Gesco International, Inc.
San Antonio, Tex.

Hill-Rom
Michael Murnane
Batesville, Ind.

IVAC Corporation
San Diego, Calif.

Instramentation Industries, Inc.
Bethel Park, Pa.

Infusaid, Inc.
A Pfizer Company
Norwood, Mass.

Kendall McGaw, Laboratories
Irvine, Calif.

3M/Medical Surgical Division
St. Paul, Minn.

Menlo Care Inc.
Palo Alto, Calif.

MiniMed Technologies
Sylmar, Calif.

Mar Tan, Inc.
Torrington, Wyo.

Northstar Laboratories, Inc.
Batavia, Ill.

Pall Biomedical Products
  Corporation
East Hills, N.Y.

Schering Corporation
Kenilworth, N.J.

Sherwood Medical Company
St. Louis, Mo.

Squibb-Novo
Princeton, N.J.

Willow Medical Home Care
  Products
Joseph Price
Springhouse, Pa.

Wyeth-Ayerst Laboratories
Division of American Home
Products Corporation
Philadelphia, Pa.

Also the staffs of:

American Red Cross
Philadelphia, Pa.

Bryn Mawr Hospital
Ann Curtis, RN
Bryn Mawr, Pa.

Chestnut Hill Hospital
Patricia Gallagher, RN
Jeffrey I. Joseph, DO
Philadelphia, Pa.

North Penn Hospital
Laurie Strauss, RN
Richard Schneider
Lansdale, Pa.

Foreword

The other day, as I walked down the hall to the unit, an older nurse in the hospital's refresher program stopped me with an urgent request: "Tell me everything I need to know about the insertion of a PICC line. My patient is having one inserted this afternoon and I'm not sure about the special care she'll need afterward." Such encounters have become increasingly common for me and other teachers of drug administration technique.

Knowing how to administer a drug correctly is as important to the nurse as knowing which drug to give and has become increasingly complex. Not only do nurses need to master a changing array of different dosage forms and complicated new equipment, they now hold a special responsibility for infection control. The critical need to prevent transmission of such dangerous infections as hepatitis and acquired immunodeficiency syndrome has led to widespread and pervasive changes in equipment and technique. So much has changed that even an expert practicing nurse needs a reliable resource at hand for checking new methods and equipment.

Such a resource is now available in a uniquely accessible form. *Photoguide to Drug Administration* provides step-by-step instruction—illustrated with clear, close up photographs—for learning virtually every drug administration procedure nurses need to know. It contains detailed, authoritative, and current instructions for giving medications correctly and safely, using everything from additive sets to Z-track injection.

An introductory section, Medication Overview, reviews the fundamental aspects of drug therapy,

including the role of the nursing process, the "seven rights" of safe drug administration (if you have been out of nursing school more than a few years, you learned only five), universal precautions, mechanisms of drug action, and guidelines for documentation and reporting.

The next section is organized by routes of administration:
• *Gastrointestinal route*—oral, tube (gastrostomy and nasogastric tubes and the gastrostomy button), and rectal administration.
• *Dermatomucosal route*—topical and mucous membrane administration.
• *Ophthalmic, otic, nasal, and laryngeal route*—ophthalmic, otic, nasal, and laryngeal administration.
• *Respiratory route*—endotracheal administration, including intermittent positive pressure breathing therapy and metered dose inhalers.

Next, a section on parenteral administration offers information on the latest equipment and techniques for injections and infusions:
• *Injection techniques*—injection equipment and intradermal, subcutaneous, and intramuscular administration.
• *Infusion techniques*—I.V. administration equipment, venipuncture, I.V. solutions, I.V. drug administration, central venous infusion, special infusion methods (intraosseous, epidural, intraventricular, and intraperitoneal), special infusion equipment, parenteral nutrition, and blood and blood product transfusion.

Valuable appendices include instruction for calculating dosages and I.V. infusion flow rates, estimating body-surface area in adults and children, an I.V. drug compatibility chart, a guide to converting units of

measure, and a list of abbreviations commonly used in medication orders.

In this unique volume, detailed instructions and clear photographs offer the reader the next best thing to seeing and touching the equipment itself. The accompanying charts and illustrations clarify complicated information. Throughout, nursing tips offer practical solutions for common problems in patient care, and include recommendations for effective patient teaching.

Photoguide to Drug Administration teaches nurses what they need to know about giving medications in clear, easy-to-read text and pictures that are truly "worth a thousand words." I enthusiastically recommend this volume not only to nursing students but also to practicing nurses in all clinical settings.

Donna M. Starsiak, RN,C, MSN
Assistant Professor of Nursing
Niehoff School of Nursing
Loyola University of Chicago

MEDICATION OVERVIEW

Reviewing Fundamentals

Administering medication in a way that ensures the patient's safety and satisfies medical and legal concerns requires meticulous attention to procedure because every route of administration carries some risk of potentially dangerous error. To help nurses meet this responsibility, the chapters that follow describe correct drug administration procedures.

This book emphasizes the importance of correct methods and techniques. However, do not overlook the fundamental importance of the nursing process, which helps direct purposeful and planned actions for patient care (see *The nursing process and drug therapy*, page 2). The nursing process provides thorough assessment, appropriate nursing diagnosis, purposeful planning, accurate implementation, and constant evaluation, which are vital for safe and effective drug administration.

Your assessment before administering a drug involves the following:
• an interview with the patient or a family member to determine which drugs the patient is currently taking
• a review of the patient's medical history and past experiences with drug administration
• a physical assessment to provide a baseline
• a review of laboratory or diagnostic test results.

Because you spend so much time with the patient, your judgment as to whether his condition is changing and a drug is no longer appropriate is often more accurate than that of other caregivers, especially when evaluations of mood and patterns of behavior are considered. Therefore, documenting your follow-up assessment of a drug's effect is critical.

Taking necessary precautions

First, identify the patient. Always check the patient's identification (wristband) before administering medication. This check allows you to care safely for responsive adults as well as for children and adults who cannot or refuse to respond correctly. Don't just rely on asking, for example, "Are you Mr. Wilson?" The patient who is not fully alert may answer yes without realizing what he is saying.

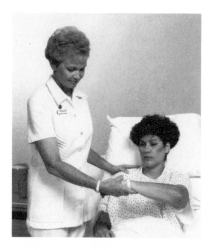

When preparing medications for administration, concentrate fully on this task and avoid distractions. Check the doctor's medication order on the patient's chart. Compare the doctor's order with the order written on the patient's medication card or Kardex, using the seven "rights" system (see *The seven "rights" of drug administration*).

Do the orders match? Double-check spelling and abbreviations to make sure you've read them correctly. Watch especially for confusing abbreviations or dangerously similar drug names, such as digoxin and digitoxin. Check the placement of the

decimal points in dosages. If you find any discrepancy, withhold the drug until you can consult the doctor. Then, correct the record and notify the supervising nurse so you can complete the appropriate incident report.

If the medication orders match the doctor's order sheet, use the seven "rights" system to check the dispensed medication against the Kardex (see *Rules of safe drug administration*, page 3).

THE SEVEN "RIGHTS" OF DRUG ADMINISTRATION

To avoid medication errors, keep the basic rules for safe drug administration in mind. Always check the doctor's order with the order written on the patient's medication card or Kardex, and remember the seven "rights" formula:
• the right drug: Is the ordered drug the same?
• the right name: Is the patient's name the same?
• the right time: Is the time and frequency of administration the same?
• the right dose: Is the ordered dose the same?
• the right route: Is the ordered route the same?
• the patient's right to know: Does the patient know why he is receiving the medication and what effects to expect?
• the patient's right to refuse medication or I.V. therapy.

THE NURSING PROCESS AND DRUG THERAPY

Safe and effective drug therapy requires understanding of a drug's action as it applies to the individual patient. This chart relates patient factors and drug factors to each step of the nursing process. Considering each factor in sequence, as listed below, promotes the best individualized nursing care during drug therapy.

PATIENT FACTORS	DRUG FACTORS

Assessment

• Physical assessment	• Completeness of drug order
• Medical history	• Appropriateness of use
• Current medical problems	• Appropriate drug route, dose, dosage form
• Emotional state	• Potential effect on laboratory findings
• Knowledge about condition and drugs	• Interactions with food or drugs
• Environment	• Institution and unit policies for drug's administration
• Allergies	
• Life-style; use of nicotine, caffeine, alcohol	

Diagnosis

• Patient problems, needs, strengths, weaknesses	• Intended use and patient response

Planning

• Plan administration taking into account patient's scheduled activities, visitors, and other medications	• Plan administration taking into account meals, patient's need for p.r.n. medications, pharmacy delivery schedule, and current supply

Interventions

• Correct and accurate drug administration	• Accurate drug preparation
• Teaching and counseling	• Safety precautions related to drug action (such as side rails up with sedatives)
• Comfort measures related to drug administration or adverse reactions	• Storage
• Observation for adverse reactions	
• Other care appropriate to condition for which drug is used, for example, wound care for patient receiving antibiotics for wound infection	
• Recording of administration	

Evaluation

• Cognitive abilities	• Therapeutic effects
• Psychomotor abilities	• Nontherapeutic effects (toxic or other adverse effects)
• Compliance factors	• Drug interactions

RULES OF SAFE DRUG ADMINISTRATION

• Be sure that you have a clear, written order for each drug administered. In an emergency, you can use a correctly documented verbal order.
• Avoid distractions when preparing and administering drugs.
• Never administer drugs taken from an unlabeled or illegibly labeled container.
• Check the medication Kardex or card against the doctor's original order to be certain that a transcription error did not occur.
• Carefully check the patient's identification band before administering any drug.
• Do not leave medication at the bedside; return any unused drug immediately to the medication area.
• Never return an unused portion of medication to a stock bottle because of the potential for returning it to the wrong bottle or contaminating the bottle.
• Do not administer medication prepared by someone else (except for unit dose forms prepared by a pharmacist). If the medication was prepared incorrectly, you would be equally responsible for the error.
• Do not prepare medication for another person to administer.
• Document all drug administration as soon as you have completed it to prevent accidental repetition of the dose by another caregiver.

Call the pharmacist if you find any discrepancy. However, don't expect the prescribed dose to match the amount on the medication label. If it doesn't, calculate how much of the medication you must give to administer the prescribed dose.

Check the Kardex for any allergies your patient may have. If the prescribed medication contains a known allergen for your patient, withhold the drug until you've consulted the doctor.

Does the dispensed medication match the information on the Kardex? Examine the drug and its container. *Never* use medication from an unlabeled container. Check the expiration or reconstitution date. Make sure the drug isn't discolored, doesn't smell unusual, and doesn't contain any precipitate (if it's a liquid). If you notice any problem or discrepancy, call the pharmacist, and return the medication to the pharmacy with an explanation. Then, place a new order.

How drugs work

When a drug enters the human body, it passes through four basic stages: absorption, distribution, metabolism, and excretion. The following information explains, in a simplified form, how each stage works.

Absorption

Absorption is the transfer of a drug from its entry site to the circulation. Common sites of drug entry are the mucosa, the GI tract, parenteral administration sites, the respiratory tract, and the skin.

Mucosa. Because the mucous membrane is the thinnest, most vascular dermal surface, drug absorption through it is fairly rapid and effective. Mucous membranes absorb drugs by diffusion, infiltration, and osmosis. The extent of absorption varies. For example, absorption through mucous membranes increases if interfering substances (such as

thick mucus in the lungs or feces in the rectum) are removed before drug administration.

GI tract. The GI tract offers the safest and easiest route for administering drugs, but drug absorption is unpredictable. Some of an orally administered drug dissolves in the stomach. The extent of dissolution depends on the size of the drug particles, the pH level of the stomach fluids, and the stomach's contents. But most of the drug is absorbed in the small intestine, which is best suited for absorption because of its large surface area, good blood supply, and pH of 6 to 8. This pH level makes most drugs nonionic, which increases lipid solubility, and promotes absorption.

Parenteral sites. Parenteral sites of administration are intradermal, subcutaneous, intramuscular, intravenous, and intra-arterial. Parenteral absorption is more reliable than GI absorption, and also more rapid. Of the five parenteral routes, the intradermal route provides the slowest absorption and is used only for very small doses. The subcutaneous route offers faster absorption than the intradermal route but slower than the intramuscular route. Subcutaneous absorption is complete.

Absorption of drugs given intramuscularly is rapid because of the large surface area and good blood supply of the muscle fibers and fasciae, but absorption may be incomplete.

Drugs given by intravenous or intra-arterial routes undergo immediate distribution throughout the patient's system because they are placed directly into the bloodstream and completely bypass absorption.

Respiratory tract. A drug is absorbed from the respiratory tract more rapidly and efficiently than from the GI tract, but more slowly than from parenteral sites. Smallparticled drugs that are inhaled are absorbed quickly from the alveoli because of the large alveolar surface area and good blood supply. The rate of absorption depends on the rate and depth of respiration and the drug's ability to cross the alveolar membrane.

Skin. Drugs that are applied to the skin for local effects are not absorbed. When a drug is applied to the skin for systemic effects, the absorption rate is determined by the density of the drug's base and the thickness of the skin where the drug is applied. Absorption through skin increases if the skin is broken, or if the area is covered and kept moist (as by an occlusive dressing) after the drug is applied. The skin may store absorbed drugs, causing photosensitivity and increasing the risk of skin damage from ultraviolet light.

Distribution

Distribution occurs when a drug binds to plasma protein in the blood and is transported via the circulation to all parts of the body, crossing cell membranes and entering body tissues. Some of the drug is distributed to and stored in fat and muscle. Release of drug from storage sites in fat and muscle can prevent a rapid decline in plasma levels as the drug is metabolized or excreted.

Metabolism

Metabolism is the conversion of a drug into a less active and more easily excreted form. Such conversion takes place mainly in the liver via synthetic and nonsynthetic reactions. In synthetic reactions, the hepatic enzymes conjugate the drug with other substances to make it less active; in nonsynthetic reactions, the drug is oxidized, hydrolyzed, and diffused. Limited metabolism also takes place in the kidneys, plasma, and intestinal mucosa. Metabolic conversion of drugs is slower in patients with hepatic disease, severe cardiovascular disease, or renal disease.

Excretion

The absorbed drug exerts an effect until it is either changed into an inactive form or is excreted. Most drugs are excreted through the kidneys, which excrete both the unchanged drug and its metabolites. They do this via passive glomerular filtration, active tubular secretion, and reabsorption. Factors affecting renal excretion are the kidneys' circulatory status, how much of the drug reaches the kidneys, and glomerular filtration rate.

Some drugs are excreted hepatically (via bile into the feces). Most drugs are excreted via the kidneys or liver, but a few may be excreted by minor routes described below:

Saliva. Drug elimination via saliva is sometimes used as an indirect index of plasma drug concentration. At a saliva pH of 5.8 to 7.1, drugs remain ionized and can't be absorbed.

Breast milk. Most drugs diffuse into the milk of a lactating woman. This may have serious implications for breast-feeding infants, for whom even a minute drug concentration may be hazardous. The amount of drug excreted in breast milk depends on the drug's lipid solubility, plasma protein binding (only free, or unbound, drug can diffuse into breast milk), and plasma drug concentration.

Sweat. Small amounts of certain drugs can sometimes be detected in sweat. Because passive diffusion dictates drug movement via sweat glands, drugs excreted by this route must be highly lipid soluble, nonionized, and non-protein bound.

Lungs. A few drugs are excreted through pulmonary alveoli via pulmonary gas exchange. For example, anesthetic gases, which usually don't undergo systemic elimination, are excreted through the lungs.

How patient factors influence drug action

Age

Patient age has a major influence on drug action because both hepatic and renal functions are altered by age extremes (immature function in neonates, and diminished function in older adults). Such patients usually require reduced drug dosages.

In elderly patients, age also influences the distribution of drugs, which is severely impaired by hardening and stiffening of blood vessels (see *Age-related changes or drug reactions?*, page 7).

Body size

Most recommended drug dosages are based on average-size adults and determined by milligrams per kilogram of body weight. Patients who are above or below average size require dosage adjustments based on body weight.

Sex

The patient's sex indirectly affects drug dosage because, on average, women are smaller than men. Also, women tend to have a higher proportion of fat cells than men; therefore, drugs that are more soluble in fat than water may be more easily distributed in women than in men. Women of childbearing age must avoid taking drugs that would be harmful to a fetus because most fetal

UNIVERSAL PRECAUTIONS

Most infectious diseases are transmitted in one of four ways: contact transmission, airborne transmission, enteric transmission, or vector-borne transmission. Infection precautions are designed to interrupt the route of transmission whereby a pathogen reaches a susceptible host.

The Centers for Disease Control (recommends the following universal precautions during the routine care of ALL patients; this means treating ALL blood and body fluids as if they're infectious.

Remember: All health care workers should routinely use appropriate barrier precautions to prevent exposure of skin and mucous membranes whenever they anticipate contact with a patient's blood or other body fluids.

ITEM	SYMBOL	PRECAUTIONS
Hands		Always wash hands before and after contact with patients, even when gloves have been worn. If hands come in contact with blood, other body fluid, or human tissue, they should be washed immediately with soap and water.
Gloves		Wear gloves whenever contact with blood, other body fluid, tissues, or contaminated surfaces is anticipated.
Gowns		Wear gowns or plastic aprons if blood splattering is likely.
Masks and goggles		Wear masks and goggles if aerosolization or splattering is likely to occur, as in certain dental and surgical procedures, wound irrigations, postmortem examinations, and bronchoscopy.
Sharp objects		Handle sharp objects carefully to prevent accidental cuts or punctures. Do not bend or break used needles, reinsert them into their original sheaths, or handle them unnecessarily. They should be discarded intact immediately after use into an impervious needle-disposal box, which should be readily accessible. All needle-stick accidents, mucosal splashes, and contamination of open wounds with blood or body fluids should be reported immediately to the department supervisor and an accident report should be filed with the employee health department.
Blood spills		Blood spills should be cleaned up promptly with an institution-designated disinfectant solution such as 5.25% sodium hypochlorite diluted 1:10 with water.
Blood specimens	DISINFECTANT	Consider all blood specimens biohazardous and label them as such.
Resuscitation		Resuscitation can involve special risk. To minimize the need for emergency mouth-to-mouth resuscitation, mouth pieces, resuscitation bags, and other ventilatory devices should be located strategically for immediate use in areas where the need for resuscitation is predictable.

damage takes place before pregnancy is identified.

Documenting medications correctly

The complete documentation of medication administration is a major nursing responsibility. Because record-keeping systems vary, you must learn the method of documentation required where you work. Whether you use medication cards, medication Kardexes, or both, you'll need the following information to complete your records: the patient's name and room number; the date; the medication; dosage; route, frequency, and time of administration; and your name and title.

Also remember the following guidelines:
• When administering a drug by the parenteral route, always record the site you selected for the injection. Doing so will make site rotation easier and will prove helpful if problems arise at the injection site. As the sample medication Kardex on pages 8 and 9 shows, some hospitals assign letters or numbers for easy site identification. Others use abbreviations for body parts, such as GM for gluteus maximus. They may also use different ink colors to distinguish between shifts.
• Never write abbreviations or numbers in a way that might confuse the other health care professionals who read your notes. For example, never abbreviate the word "unit". Someone may misread the letter "U" for a poorly written zero and administer an incorrect dose. To clearly show doses that contain fractions of grams, put a 0 *before* the decimal point, as in 0.25 mg digoxin. Then no one will misread it for 25 mg.
• After giving a medication, document it as soon as possible. If a drug was ordered but not given, note this on the Kardex, and chart the reason

why in your nurse's notes. When you give a medication that's to be administered when needed, such as an analgesic, chart why it was given, whether or not it proved effective, and if it caused any adverse reaction.
• If a patient's drug regimen is discontinued because surgery has been scheduled, be sure to indicate this.

Documenting oral orders

A written drug order, signed by a doctor, provides all the legal authority you require to administer a drug without incurring liability. However, an oral (spoken) order, whether given to you in person or by telephone, requires the following steps for protection from legal liability:

1 Write down the order exactly as the prescribing doctor gives it.

2 Repeat the order to the prescribing doctor as you received it to confirm that you heard the order correctly.

3 After administering the drug, make sure you document all necessary information.

Record in ink the name of the drug, the dose, the time you administered it, and any other information your institution's policy requires. Sign or initial your notes.

If your institution keeps drug orders in a special file, be sure to transfer the doctor's drug order, which you wrote on the patient's chart, to that file.

If a doctor gives you a drug order during an emergency, consider that such an oral order can be carried out only by a registered nurse. Always repeat the name of the medication, dosage, route of administration, and patient's name. When the emergency is over, document what you did and have the doctor countersign the order.

Severe liability

Consider the grave consequences that can follow if you fail to document oral orders correctly: You could face disciplinary measures for failing to document.

You could damage your institution's defense of your defense in any malpractice lawsuit. If undocumented drug administration is uncovered in a malpractice suit, it is called negligence. Also, other nurses, not knowing which drugs the patient has already received, may administer additional drugs that could have harmful consequences.

Safeguarding against errors

Keep in mind the following safeguards against giving the wrong drug:
• Avoid distractions during preparation and administration.
• Separate look-alike medications, and separate medications from toxic chemicals.
• Discard outdated drugs.
• Don't administer medications with unapproved abbreviations.
• Check labels and package inserts to know the peculiarities and dangers of a drug before giving it.
• Read and follow warnings on drug labels.
• Always check with the pharmacy if any doubts arise.

Observe these safeguards against giving a drug by the wrong route:
• Use only accepted injection sites.
• Aspirate before giving an I.M. injection.
• Choose and use the right length needle.

Questioning drug orders

When in doubt about the appropriateness of a drug order, follow your institution's policy when questioning it. Usually, the policy suggests pursuing the following steps in the sequence listed until you obtain a satisfactory answer:

AGE-RELATED CHANGES OR DRUG REACTIONS?

Many drugs can cause signs often attributed to age-related changes, such as confusion and forgetfulness. The chart below lists drugs (or drug combinations) that may cause such signs. Drug-related signs can often be relieved by dosage adjustment.

SIGNS	POSSIBLE CAUSES
Anorexia	Digoxin (Lanoxin)
Ataxia	Phenytoin (Dilantin), high doses or prolonged use of flurazepam (Dalmane) and other sedatives or hypnotics
Confusion	Methyldopa (Aldomet), digoxin, cimetidine (Tagamet)
Constipation	Medications with anticholinergic properties, such as belladonna-containing drugs; narcotics; tricyclic antidepressants; iron preparations
Depression	Reserpine (Serpasil)
Diarrhea	Antacid preparations containing magnesium, quinidine (Duraquin)
Forgetfulness	Barbiturates, methyldopa
Lethargy and drowsiness	Various antianxiety agents, analgesics, antihistamines, sedatives, and hypnotics, including chlorpromazine (Thorazine) and pentobarbital (Nembutal)
Tremor	Antipsychotics, cerebral stimulants, antidepressants
Weakness	Potassium-wasting diuretics, such as furosemide (Lasix) and hydrochlorothiazide (Esidrix)
Urine retention	Antipsychotics, antidepressants

• Look up the answer in a standard drug reference.
• Ask the charge nurse.
• Ask the pharmacist.
• Ask the prescribing doctor.
• Ask the prescribing doctor's supervisor (service chief).

Refusing to administer a drug

You have the legal right not to administer a drug you have reason to believe will be harmful to a patient. You may exercise this right when:
• you believe the prescribed dose is incorrect and this is verified by the pharmacy.
• you believe the drug is contraindicated because of possible dangerous interactions with other drugs or with other substances, such as alcohol.
• your assessment of the patient's physical condition contraindicates use of the drug.

In limited circumstances, you may also legally refuse to administer a drug on grounds of conscience. Some states and provinces have enacted right-of-conscience laws that excuse medical personnel from the requirement to participate in any abortion or sterilization procedure. Under such laws, you may, for example, refuse to give any drug you believe is intended to induce abortion.

When you refuse to carry out a drug order, be sure to:

• notify your immediate supervisor so she can make alternative arrangements (assigning a new nurse, clarifying the order)
• notify the prescribing doctor if your supervisor hasn't done so
• document that the drug was not given and explain why (keep in mind, however, that a supervisor, doctor, or another nurse may give the drug).

Preparing an incident report

If you make an error in giving a drug, or if a patient reacts adversely to a properly administered drug, you must document the incident to protect yourself from liability. Some of the required documentation belongs

(Text continues on page 10.)

SAMPLE MEDICATION KARDEX

Allergic To: _Penicillin_
(record in red)

Dates Given _____   Date Discharged _____

Date	Medication, Dose Frequency	Hr.	1/31																
1/31	Inderal 10 mg po Q 6°	12^{M}	BW																
		6^{A}	BW																
		12^{N}	HN																
		6^{P}	KC																
1/31	Demerol 50 mg IM Q 4° PRN { chest pain unrelieved { by Ntg X2	11-7	2P/ BW LD																
		7-3																	
		3-11																	
1/31	Ntg. gr 1/150 SL PRN chest pain	11-7	1:30A/ BW 1:45A/ BW																
		7-3																	
		3-11																	

AGE **62**   RELIGION **J**   DATE ADMITTED **1/31/91**   DOCTOR **Rose** _____   INTERN _____

NAME _David Bernard_ _____   ROOM **203**   DIAGNOSIS _Unstable Angina_ _____

Date	Time	No.	Problem	Nursing Action and Patient Outcome
1/31	1:30/A	1	chest pain	A: diaphoretic, BP 160/100 apical R-132, resp 28, lungs clear I: MD notified. O2 applied @ 2L/min as ordered, Ntg gr 1/150 SL given BW
	1:45/A			A: pain unrelieved BP 160/110, apical R 140, resp 24 I: Ntg gr 1/150 SL repeated BW
	2/A			A: pain continues BP 150/110 apical R 120, resp 24 I: ECG done, Demerol 50 mg given BW
	2:20/A			O: pain relieved, pt resting comfortably, BP 130/190 apical R 88, resp 20 Bonnie Weaver, RN

ABBREVIATIONS

LA: Left Abdomen   **RA:** Right Abdomen   **LT:** Left Thigh   **RT:** Right Thigh   **LD:** Left Deltoid
LB: Left Buttock   **RB:** Right Buttock   **O:** Patient Outcome   **A:** Assessment   **I:** Intervention

in the patient's chart, including information on the patient's reaction and any medical or nursing interventions taken to minimize harm to the patient. Other documentation should be confined to the formal incident report, which is required by federal agencies and the Joint Commission on Accreditation of Healthcare Organizations. On the incident report form (see sample), you must objectively identify what happened, the names and functions of all persons involved, and the actions taken to protect the patient after the error was discovered.

An incident report does not become part of the patient's medical record, nor does it replace nursing documentation in the patient's chart. The patient's medical record should not mention that an incident report has been filed, but should include objective clinical observations relating to the incident (subjective judgments must be avoided). Entering observations about the incident in the patient's record, however, does not replace the requirement for completing an incident report.

An incident report explains the circumstances as they existed and the safeguards you took to make your actions safe. It demonstrates that despite all precautions, an error or injury occurred.

The incident report serves two main purposes:
• to inform supervisors about the incident so they can consider changes that will help prevent similar incidents (risk management)
• to alert administrators and the institution's insurance company to potential liability claims and the need for further investigation (claims management).

Even when the incident is not investigated, the report helps to identify witnesses in case of a future lawsuit.

WHAT TO DO IF A PATIENT REFUSES MEDICATION

Never force a patient to take medication. If a patient refuses a medication, try to find out why. After you explain what the medication is and its purpose, the patient will usually take the dose.

If the patient still refuses, report this to the charge nurse and the doctor, and record the patient's reason for refusing the medication in your nurse's notes. Discard the medication, except any that was dispensed in a unit dose system. In the latter case, return the medication in its wrapper or container, with appropriate documentation, to the pharmacy.

Only a person with firsthand knowledge of an incident should report it, and only the reporting person should sign it. Each person with firsthand knowledge should fill out and sign a separate report. Never sign a report describing circumstances or events that you have not witnessed personally.

A patient-related incident report should include only the following:
• the identities of the patient and any witnesses
• information about what happened and how it affected the patient (supply enough objective information so that administrators can decide if the matter needs further investigation, but omit evaluation and commentary).

Because nursing supervisors try to identify causes of such incidents, there's a tendency to include evaluation and opinion. Remember that subjective information should be excluded from the body of the report and be placed in the narrative section. The incident report serves only

to notify the administration that an incident has occurred. In effect it says, "Administration: Note that this incident happened, and decide if further investigation is warranted." Such items as detailed statements from witnesses and descriptions of remedial action are normally part of an investigative follow-up and should not be included in the report.

Each institution has specific policies and procedures for filing incident reports. It's your duty as a licensed professional to know your institution's policy.

INCIDENT REPORT

HOSPITAL NAME	HOSPITAL CODE NO.	DEPARTMENT OR STATION	SHIFT SUPERVISOR	SHIFT ☐ FIRST ☐ THIRD ☐ SECOND

NAME OF PARTY INVOLVED IN INCIDENT		DATE OF THIS REPORT	TIME OF INCIDENT	DATE OF INCIDENT
last	first		☐ A.M. ☐ P.M.	

ADDRESS		SEX	ADMITTING DX(IF PATIENT)
street	city state	☐ MALE ☐ FEMALE	

IDENTIFICATION 1 ☐ INPATIENT 3 ☐ ED PATIENT 5 ☐ EMPLOYEE   AGE   EXACT LOCATION OF INCIDENT
                2 ☐ OUTPATIENT 4 ☐ VISITOR 6 ☐ OTHER

AREA INCIDENT OCCURED 1 ☐ OPERATING ROOM 3 ☐ PATIENT ROOM 5 ☐ INTENSIVE CARE UNIT 7 ☐ PARKING LOT
                       2 ☐ EMERGENCY ROOM 4 ☐ PATIENT BATHROOM 6 ☐ HOSPITAL GROUNDS 8 ☐ OTHER (SPECIFY)_____

TO BE COMPLETED BY DOCTOR

NATURE OF INJURY
1 ☐ CONTUSION, CUT, LACERATION   6 ☐ VISCERA INJURY   10 ☐ OTHER (SPECIFY)
2 ☐ FRACTURE, DISLOCATION   7 ☐ SPRAIN, STRAIN   _____
3 ☐ NEEDLE WOUND   8 ☐ BURN, SCALD   _____
4 ☐ CHEMICAL BURN   9 ☐ NO APPARENT INJURY   _____
5 ☐ CONCUSSION

DATE NOTIFIED: DATE PATIENT EXAMINED:
TIME NOTIFIED: TIME PATIENT EXAMINED:

EXAMINATION FINDINGS: _____

DOCTOR NAME: DOCTOR NAME:

DOCUMENTED IN PROGRESS NOTE ☐

DISPOSITION

SEEN BY	TREATMENT	NOTIFICATION (Check all applicable boxes)	NAME	DATE AND TIME
1 ☐ ATTENDING PHYSICIAN	1 ☐ X-RAY ORDERED	1 ☐ YES 1 ☐ NO UNIT	_____	_____
2 ☐ EMERGENCY DEPT.	2 ☐ ADMITTED TO HOSPITAL	2 ☐ YES 2 ☐ NO NOTED IN CHART	_____	_____
3 ☐ OTHER (SPECIFY)	3 ☐ TREATMENT RENDERED	3 ☐ YES 3 ☐ NO PRIVATE (ATTENDING DOCTOR)	_____	_____
_____		4 ☐ YES 4 ☐ NO SECURITY	_____	_____
		5 ☐ YES 5 ☐ NO ADMINISTRATION	_____	_____
	4 ☐ FOLLOW-UP CARE INDICATED	6 ☐ YES 6 ☐ NO SUPERVISOR	_____	_____

CONDITION BEFORE INCIDENT 1 ☐ SEDATED 3 ☐ UNKNOWN
                           2 ☐ UNCONSCIOUS 4 ☐ OTHER(SPECIFY)_____

NATURE OF INCIDENT (Check only one)

FALL
1 WHILE INSIDE BUILDING
2 WHILE OUTSIDE BUILDING
3 WHILE SITTING
4 OUT OF BED
5 OFF TABLE OR EQUIPMENT
6 OTHER (SPECIFY)_____

BURN
1 ☐ ELECTRICITY
2 ☐ HEATING APPLIANCE
3 ☐ SPILL
4 ☐ CIGARETTE, CIGAR, ETC.
5 ☐ OTHER (SPECIFY)_____

MEDICATION
1 ☐ ERROR IN PATIENT IDENTIFICATION
2 ☐ INCORRECT DRUG
3 ☐ INCORRECT DOSAGE
4 ☐ MODE OF ADMINISTRATION
5 ☐ TIMING
6 ☐ DUPLICATION
7 ☐ OMISSION
8 ☐ BLOOD TRANSFUSION
9 ☐ NAME OF MEDICATION
10 ☐ OTHER (SPECIFY)_____

ARTICLE IN PATIENT
1 ☐ NEEDLE
2 ☐ INSTRUMENT
3 ☐ SPONGE
4 ☐ OTHER (SPECIFY)_____

PATIENT INDUCED
1 ☐ ATTEMPTED SUICIDE
2 ☐ INFLICTED BY OTHER PATIENT
3 ☐ AMA ABSENCE

MISCELLANEOUS I
1 ☐ GENERAL POWER FAILURE
2 ☐ ELEVATOR RELATED
3 ☐ STRUCK BY DOOR
4 ☐ FIRE
5 ☐ FLOOD

MISCELLANEOUS II
1 ☐ INJECTION
2 ☐ PATIENT IDENTIFICATION
3 ☐ INJURIES IN TREATMENT
4 ☐ INFECTION
5 ☐ I.V. TECHNIQUES
6 ☐ ELECTRICAL SHOCK
7 ☐ ENTERING/EXITING BUILDING
8 ☐ EQUIPMENT (DESCRIBE)_____
9 ☐ OTHER (SPECIFY)_____

PATIENT VALUABLES	ARTICLES DESCRIBED	AMBULATION PRIVILEGES	SIDE RAILS (Three Quarter)
1 ☐ DAMAGED	1 ☐ DENTURES _____	1 ☐ COMPLETE BED REST 5 ☐ NOT SPECIFIED	1 ☐ ONE UP
2 ☐ LOST	2 ☐ EYE GLASSES _____	2 ☐ BED REST WITH BRP 6 ☐ OTHER (SPECIFY)	2 ☐ ON BED NOT UP
3 ☐ OTHER (SPECIFY)	3 ☐ HEARING AID _____	3 ☐ OOB WITH ASSISTANCE _____	3 ☐ TWO UP
_____	4 ☐ JEWELRY _____	4 ☐ OOB	
	5 ☐ OTHER (SPECIFY)_____		

SIDE RAILS (Half Rails)	RESTRAINTS PRESENT	RESTRAINTS ORDERED	BED HEIGHT
1 ☐ ONE UP 4 ☐ FOUR UP	1 ☐ YES	1 ☐ YES	1 ☐ HIGH POSTION
2 ☐ TWO UP 5 ☐ ON BED, NOT UP	2 ☐ NO	2 ☐ NO	2 ☐ LOW POSITION
3 ☐ THREE UP			

NARRATIVE DESCRIPTION OF INCIDENT, INCLUDING STATEMENT OF PARTY INVOLVED: _____
☐ IF MORE SPACE IS NEEDED PLEASE CHECK BOX AND CONTINUE ON ADDITIONAL PAGE

WITNESS ☐ YES ☐ NO   IF YES, COMPLETE THE FOLLOWING

WITNESS (INCLUDING ADDRESS)

last	first	street	city	state	zip

PERSON COMPLETING FORM	REVIEWED BY SHIFT SUPERVISOR
PRINT NAME TITLE	PRINT NAME TITLE
SIGNATURE DATE	SIGNATURE DATE

GASTROINTESTINAL ROUTE

Oral Administration

Oral administration provides the most convenient and least expensive method of introducing medication into the body and is the most commonly used route for many drugs. Solid oral forms include tablets, capsules, extended release tablets or capsules, and enteric (coated) tablets or capsules. Liquid forms include syrups, elixirs, emulsions, and suspensions (see *Reviewing liquid oral medications,* page 17).

How oral medication is absorbed

After ingestion, solid tablets and capsules disintegrate and dissolve in either the stomach or the small intestine. Because liquids do not undergo this transformation, they may be absorbed more rapidly and completely than tablets or capsules and reach peak serum concentration levels more rapidly.

Several factors may influence the dissolution rate of solid medication: particle size, pH, gastric emptying and peristaltic rate, and the effect of ingested foods and beverages.

Particle size

Chewable tablets dissolve more quickly than those swallowed whole; small particles usually dissolve in the gastric fluids more readily than large particles. The type and amount of filler (inert substances) contained in the tablet or capsule also influence the dissolution rate.

pH

Acidic medications are more soluble in the alkaline fluids of the small intestine; alkaline medications are more soluble in the acidic fluids of the stomach.

Gastric emptying and peristaltic rate

Various factors influence the rate of gastric emptying, including the patient's hormonal activity, physical activity, and the volume, temperature, and pH of the stomach contents. Body position can also influence gastric emptying. To encourage gastric emptying, position the patient upright or on the right side. To slow gastric emptying (for example, to prolong the effects of an antacid in the stomach), position the patient on the left side to keep the medication in the stomach longer.

An increased peristaltic rate, such as from diarrhea, can decrease absorption by moving the medication through the small intestine too rapidly.

Foods and beverages

Whether medication should be given with meals or between meals depends on the medication. Food can protect the gastric mucosa from drug irritation, but a full stomach can slow the absorption rate or change the drug's therapeutic effects. For example, some penicillins decompose prematurely when mixed with fruit juices. Griseofulvin (Grisactin) is absorbed completely only in the presence of fatty food.

Dilution with a beverage such as fruit juice can enhance absorption if the medication and the beverage are compatible. Therefore, it's always important to check for such incompatibilities before administering any medication.

Learning about tablets and capsules

Tablets come in various sizes, shapes, and colors. In addition to the drug

HOW ORAL MEDICATION IS ABSORBED IN THE G.I. TRACT

The illustration below compares the various sites of dissolution, disintegration, and absorption for different forms of orally administered drugs.

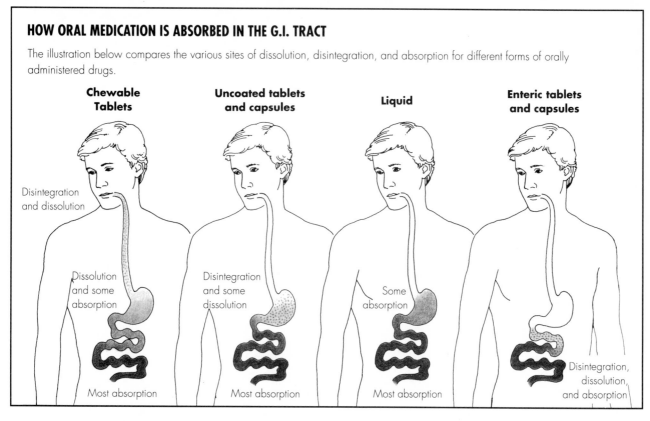

Chewable Tablets
Disintegration and dissolution
Dissolution and some absorption
Most absorption

Uncoated tablets and capsules
Disintegration and some dissolution
Most absorption

Liquid
Some absorption
Most absorption

Enteric tablets and capsules
Disintegration, dissolution, and absorption

itself, tablets may contain one or more of the following ingredients:

• diluents, such as lactose, starch, or dextrose, to add bulk and ensure correct size and consistency

• disintegrants, such as starch, to speed dissolution

• coatings, to add color, disguise an unpleasant taste, protect the gastric mucosa from irritation, and protect the tablet from light, air, and moisture. An enteric coating allows the tablet to pass through the stomach intact and dissolve in the duodenum, where the drug is absorbed.

Some uncoated tablets are scored for easy division into halves or quarters, if the dose calls for only a portion of the tablet.

Like tablets, capsules come in various colors, shapes, and sizes, ranging from ½" to 1" (1.2 cm to 2.5 cm). Capsules may contain powders, granules, gels, oils, or other liquids. Some capsules contain particles of medica-

tion that have been coated with substances that permit controlled release of the medication over a prolonged period. Most capsules have thin gelatin shells; some have shells of harder gelatin or enteric coatings. Because capsules contain medication in particle or liquid form, it's usually absorbed faster than medication in a compressed tablet.

Both tablets and capsules may be packaged as single unit doses in foil or cellophane blister packs, as shown.

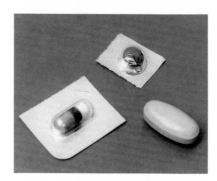

How to give tablets and capsules

Before administering any medication, double check the medication label and compare it to the doctor's order. Confirm the patient's identity by checking the wristband. Assess the patient's condition. For example, you may want to withhold a medication that will slow the patient's heart rate if the patient's apical pulse rate is below 60 beats/minute. Then proceed as follows:

1 Wash your hands thoroughly, and remember to maintain clean technique throughout the procedure. Gather the equipment. If you plan to crush a tablet, you'll need a mortar and pestle or a commercially made pulverizer; to divide a scored tablet, you'll need a knife. Usually, all you need is the bottle of medication, a small souffle cup or medicine cup, and water or juice.

2 Pour the correct number of tablets or capsules into the bottle cap. If you pour out too many, put the excess back.

Never touch any of the excess medication or you may contaminate the entire bottle. For the same reason, don't return the unused portion of a divided tablet to the bottle; discard it.

3 Pour the tablets or capsules into the souffle cup or medicine cup, and recap the medication bottle. Then give the cup to the patient or tap the medication into his hand. Keep the water or juice nearby. Stay with the patient until he has swallowed the drug.

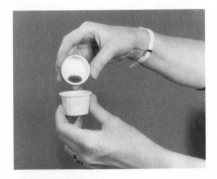

NURSING TIP If the patient has trouble swallowing tablets or capsules, have him drink some water before taking the medication.

4 Tell the patient to put the tablets or capsules well back on the tongue. He may take them one at a time or all at once, whichever he prefers. If he can't do this himself, put on gloves and administer the medication, as shown.

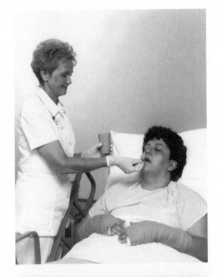

Avoid touching the patient's mouth or the rim of the medication cup after the patient has used it. If you do, wash your hands immediately to avoid transferring bacteria to your next patient.

5 Ask the patient to tip his head slightly forward, and swallow a mouthful of water or juice. Warn the patient not to throw his head back as he swallows. This position may prevent the airway from closing and may increase the risk of aspiration. Finally, discard the used souffle cup and document the procedure.

How to measure liquid medication in a disposable cup

1 After you confirm the doctor's order, wash your hands, and identify and assess the patient, you're ready to measure the prescribed dose of liquid oral medication.

ADMINISTERING ORAL DRUGS

Advantages
● Administration is simple and convenient. Usually, the patient can self-administer the drug.
● In case of overdose, gastric lavage or induced vomiting may dilute or retrieve the drug before it can cause toxic effects.

Disadvantages
● Relatively slow absorption rate makes the oral route unsuitable for most emergencies.
● Because the amount of drug that reaches the patient's circulation varies depending on the extent of absorption in the patient's GI tract, the effectiveness of an oral drug is somewhat unpredictable.
● Some oral drugs irritate the GI tract. Others can discolor the teeth.
● Oral drugs are not suitable for all patients. For example, patients who are combative or severely debilitated, or who have a history of drug abuse usually should not receive oral drugs. Oral drugs can be particularly hazardous in households that include small children, unless the drugs are stored safely out of the children's reach.

To begin, you'll need the bottle of medication, a disposable medicine cup, and a damp paper towel. If you plan to dilute the medication, obtain some water or juice (make sure the medication's compatible with the diluent).

Choose a disposable medicine cup that has all the markings you need. Never try to estimate measurements *between* markings or the dose won't be accurate. Check the bottle label against the Kardex.

If the medication is a suspension, shake it well. Then, uncap the bottle and place the cap upside down on a clean surface.

Rinse the medication cup in water. This will prevent medication from sticking to its sides.

2 Locate the correct marking on the medicine cup. Keeping thumbnail on the mark, hold the cup at eye level, as shown, and pour the correct amount of medication.

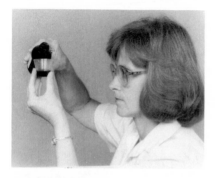

NURSING TIP   As you pour, keep the label pointed up so spills won't obscure it. Recheck the label against the Kardex. If you've poured too much medication into the cup, dis-card the excess. Don't return it to the bottle.

3 Wipe the bottle lip with a damp paper towel, taking care not to touch the side of the bottle. Replace the cap. Recheck the label against the Kardex.

4 Position the patient comfortably in either a sitting or high Fowler's position. Hand her the cup of medication, and wait until she drinks it all.

Discard the medicine cup, taking care not to touch the rim. Finally, document the entire procedure.

How to give medication to an infant

Any oral medication you administer to an infant will be liquid and prescribed in very small doses. Use a dropper to ensure accuracy. Here's how:

1 Put a bib under the infant's chin and a diaper or towel over your shoulder. Then, position the infant in the crook of your arm. Hold him so his head is elevated at a 45-degree angle. If necessary, use one of your hands to restrain his arms.

2 With your other hand, withdraw the correct amount of medication from the bottle by squeezing the bulb on the dropper.

If the dropper's calibrated, check the dose by holding it vertically and looking at it from eye level. Squeeze any excess into a sink or wastebasket. Don't return it to the bottle.

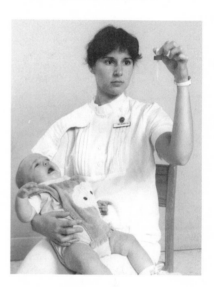

NURSING CONSIDERATIONS: ORAL ADMINISTRATION

To help some patients swallow tablets or capsules, you may crush uncoated tablets or open soft uncoated capsules and then mix the medication in a small amount of a compatible beverage or food, such as applesauce or mashed potatoes. Always make sure the mixture won't change the drug's action. Because the medication may change the taste of the food or beverage, be sure to tell the patient what you've done.

• Never crush or open coated tablets or capsules or hard capsules. Destroying such coatings will prevent proper absorption of the medication.
• Administer coated tablets and capsules with plenty of water when the patient's stomach is empty to ensure quick passage into the small intestine. Tell the patient not to chew coated tablets or capsules, but to swallow them whole.
• Opening sustained-release cap-sules may alter the dose. The microbeads of medication in such capsules have coatings of varying thicknesses that are designed to dissolve over 12 to 24 hours.
• Protect tablets and capsules from light, humidity, and air. Signs of deterioration include discoloration and unusual odor. Return any medication that looks or smells strange to the pharmacy.
• Check the expiration date and discard any outdated medication.

3 Get ready to instill the drops. If the infant won't open his mouth, try pinching his cheeks gently.

If the dropper's not calibrated, hold it vertically over the infant's open mouth, and instill the prescribed number of drops.

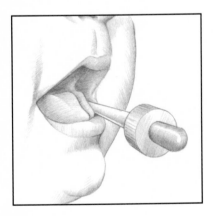

If you're using a calibrated dropper, instill the medication into the pocket between the infant's cheek and his gum. Putting the medication in that spot will keep him from spitting it out and reduces the risk of aspiration.

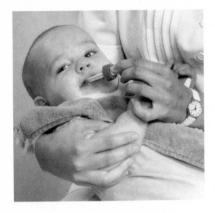

4 If the dropper touches the inside of the infant's mouth, consider it contaminated. Wash the dropper thoroughly with soap and water; then, rinse and dry it.

Suppose you've prevented contamination. If the dropper's attached to the bottle cap, simply return it to the bottle and screw the cap on tight-

ly. But if it's unattached, rinse the medication out of it with warm water, put it in a clean plastic bag, and store it with the infant's medication bottle. Document the procedure.

> Never use the same dropper for more than one patient. Keep each infant's dropper separate and labeled with his name. Dispose of the dropper when the medication's gone.

Giving medication to special patients

Children
A school-age child can probably swallow a tablet or capsule safely, but may be more willing to take a sweet-tasting syrup or chewable tablet. Avoid problems by finding out if the medication's available in either of these forms. Avoid giving a child an elixir because he'll probably dislike the alcohol flavor. But if you must, dilute it first with a small amount of water.

Encourage the child's cooperation by acting as if you expect it. However, if he balks, don't threaten or embarrass him. Never insist that he swallow a medication. Doing so may cause him to aspirate.

When giving medication to a child, keep these pointers in mind:
• Avoid mixing medication with food. The child who detects a strange taste may refuse that particular food in the future.
• When you know medication will taste bad, say so. Don't try to trick a child. Doing so will make him less cooperative next time.
• Never tell a child that medication's candy. He may look for an opportu-

nity to eat or drink the entire contents of the bottle.
• Praise the child for cooperation, if you get it. Let him keep the medicine cup as a trophy, but be sure to rinse it out first.
• Enlist support from the child's parents.

Stroke patients
If the patient's ability to swallow is seriously impaired, giving oral medication isn't safe. But what if he's a stroke patient and only one side of his head and body is affected? If he's alert and cooperative, with your help he may be able to swallow oral medication.

Before you begin, remember that your patient's stroke has probably affected him in many ways. Keep this in mind when you give him his medication. For example, if the vision on his impaired side is affected, approach and treat him from his unimpaired side so he can see what you're doing. If he suffers from some form of aphasia, speak to him slowly, explaining the procedure in words he can understand. Don't bombard him with information or you may confuse him. Speak calmly and reassuringly.

To determine if a patient can swallow effectively, have him sit in a high Fowler's position. Fill a glass three-quarters full with water (no straw), then have the patient take some water, tilt his head back, and then swallow. If the patient has a delayed or absent swallowing reflex, he will choke on the water.

Try to give the medication in solid form, because a textured substance is easier to control than a liquid for such a patient. Crush uncoated tablets or open soft capsules, and mix them with a soft foods such as applesauce or mashed potatoes. However, never mix the medication with a milk product. Milk products will stimulate

REVIEWING LIQUID ORAL MEDICATIONS

TYPE AND DESCRIPTION	NURSING CONSIDERATIONS
Syrup	
A drug and preservative in a viscous sugar and water solution; usually flavored	• When giving a syrup (for example, cough syrup) for a demulcent (soothing) effect, don't follow it with water. Tell the patient to sip the syrup slowly. • When giving a syrup for a systemic effect, you may dilute it. However, dilute only the dose being given. If you dilute the entire bottle, you may destroy the preservative and hasten contamination or decomposition. • Use caution when administering syrups to diabetic patients. Check with the pharmacist to see if a sugar-free syrup is available. • When giving syrups with other drugs, be sure to administer syrups last. • Take special care to keep syrups out of children's reach.
Suspension	
Magma: thick, milky suspension of an insoluble (or partly soluble) inorganic drug suspended in water *Gel:* the same as magma but with smaller drug particles *Emulsion:* droplets of fat or oil suspended in water	• Always shake a suspension thoroughly before giving it. • If desired, you may dilute most suspensions with water before administration. Don't dilute an antacid suspension, or it won't coat the stomach effectively.
Solution with alcohol	
Elixir: clear, sweet-tasting mixture of a drug, alcohol, water, and sugar. Elixirs are less sweet and less viscous than syrups. Alcohol concentration ranges from 8% to 78%. *Spirits:* solution of volatile substances, such as liquids, solids, or gases. The alcohol in the solution acts as a preservative and solvent. The solution is used primarily as a flavoring agent. *Tincture:* a solution of alcohol, or alcohol and water, with animal or vegetable products or chemical substances *Fluidextract:* bitter solution of vegetable drugs, usually sweetened with a syrup or flavoring. Fluidextracts are rarely prescribed because they are unusually potent as well as unpleasant tasting. The alcohol in the solution acts as a solvent or a preservative, or both.	• Check the solution carefully. Never administer one that contains precipitate at the bottom of the bottle. • If you want to dilute the solution, use only a small amount of water. Too much water could cause the drug to precipitate. • Consult the pharmacist before you mix solutions containing alcohol with liquids other than water. Mixing with other liquids may be contraindicated. • Follow administration with water, unless the solution's given to relieve cough. • Store solution in an airtight container. Protect from temperature extremes. • Do not administer such solutions to a known alcoholic. Use caution if you suspect that the patient abuses alcohol. • Never give a solution containing alcohol to a patient who is receiving disulfiram (Antabuse). • Use extreme caution when administering such solutions to elderly patients. Request alcohol-free solutions for patients who have had adverse reactions in the past.
Reconstituted powders and tablets	
Solid drugs reconstituted with water (or another suitable liquid) and given to the patient in suspension or solution form	• Read the directions carefully before reconstituting powders and tablets. Don't use too much water with effervescent tablets or they'll boil out of the glass. • Some powders become gelatinous very quickly after mixing. Administer them immediately after reconstitution. • Wait until effervescent tablets dissolve completely before you give them to the patient. Then give without further dilution.

salivation, which will increase the risk of aspiration.

Minimize the risk of aspiration in any stroke patient by following this procedure:

• When you're giving him medication or food, put it on the back of his tongue on the *unimpaired* side of his mouth. Then, gently turn his head toward the unimpaired side and tilt the head forward.

Never tilt a stroke patient's head backward. This position makes aspiration more likely.

• Give him a sip of water, and ask him to swallow. At the same time press lightly on the *impaired* side of his neck, to stimulate the swallowing reflex. Continue to give him small sips of water until he's swallowed the food or medication. Then, check his mouth. Remove any food or medication trapped on his impaired side.

• Finally, document the entire procedure. Record foods that seem to give your patient particular trouble. For example, if he has difficulty swallowing applesauce, make a note on his care plan and medication Kardex not to mix his medication with applesauce.

As always, assess the patient at each medication time. If you think giving oral medication's too risky for your patient, tell the doctor. He may choose another route.

NURSING TIP   If your patient's afraid of choking on his medication, place the fingers of his unimpaired hand on his neck. When he feels his neck muscles working as he swallows, his confidence may be restored. To be perfectly safe, however, have suctioning equipment handy.

Patients with tracheostomies

Be especially careful when you're giving medication to a patient with a tracheostomy tube.

• Suction the tracheostomy and make sure the cuff's inflated, because the inflated cuff blocks off the trachea around the outer cannula, preventing aspiration. However, if the patient has a trach-talk attachment, replace it with a one-piece trach tube and inflate the cuff or he won't be able to exhale.

• Don't rush when you give the medication. If the patient coughs or chokes, stop what you're doing immediately. Then wait until he's calm before you continue.

• Tell the doctor if the patient had difficulty swallowing the medication.

• Have the patient sit upright.

• Never administer large tablets or capsules.

• Document the entire procedure.

Tube Administration

Medication can be instilled through a nasogastric (NG) tube or through a surgically placed gastrostomy tube. Drug action is the same as with oral administration; however, the drug must be in liquid form or crushed and well dissolved just before administration.

How to insert an NG tube

Identify the patient, assess her condition, and plan modifications if necessary. Then proceed as follows:

1 Wash your hands and gather the equipment shown. Follow these guidelines for determining NG tube size: for an infant, #6 to #8 French; for an older child, #8 to #12 French; and for an adult, #12 to #18 French. Test the tube's patency by running water through it. Examine it for rough or ragged edges.

NURSING TIP Because most NG tubes are now made of vinyl, the one you choose may be too stiff to insert gently. If it is, you can increase its flexibility by dipping it in warm water for several minutes. If you're using a rubber tube that's too flexible to maneuver easily during insertion, chill the tube with ice to give it the rigidity you need.

2 Provide privacy for your patient. Next, tell the patient what you're about to do in words she can understand. Answer any questions. To give a sense of control during this uncomfortable procedure, agree on a signal that will tell you to wait for a moment, such as raising her hand or tapping your arm. Then, place her in a comfortable upright position, either sitting or in a high Fowler's position, as shown. Protect her gown and the bed from spills with bedsaver pads and a towel. Offer plenty of tissues because intubation may stimulate tearing. Hand her the emesis basin in case she vomits.

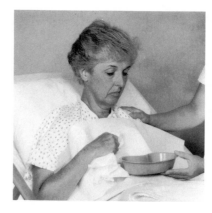

Now, use a penlight to check her nostrils for possible obstruction. Then, alternately press each of her nostrils shut, and ask her to inhale through the open nostril. Choose the more patent of the two nostrils for insertion. If neither is patent, notify the doctor.

3 Use this simple two-step method to determine how much tube to insert. First, measure the distance

EQUIPMENT FOR N.G. TUBE INSERTION

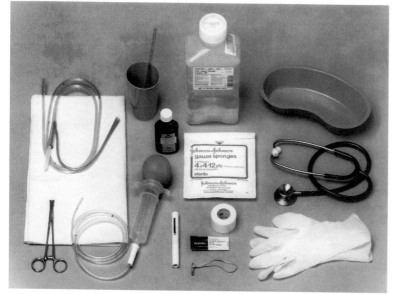

Nasogastric tube with pigtail	Cup with straw	Normal saline solution	Emesis basin
Bedsaver pad	Tincture of benzoin	4" x 4" gauze pad	Stethoscope
Hemostat	Bulb syringe with Levin nasogastric tube	Tape	Gloves
	Pen light	Water-soluble lubricant	
		Safety pin and rubber band	

from the patient's earlobe to the bridge of her nose, as shown.

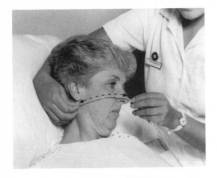

Then, measure from the bridge of her nose to the bottom of her xiphoid process. Total these figures, and mark the desired length on the tube with adhesive tape.

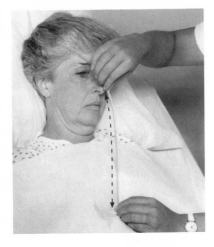

To measure an infant or child, turn his head to one side. Then, measure the distance from the tip of his nose to his earlobe; then from his earlobe to a point midway between the xiphoid process and the umbilicus. Total these measurements, and mark the tube.

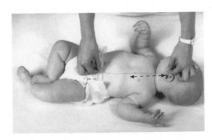

4 When the tube is marked, hold it 6" to 8" (15.2 to 20.3 cm) from the tips. Roll it between your fingers to find the natural curve. If necessary, shape a curve yourself by coiling the first 5" (12.7 cm) around your fingers. Lubricate the first 6" of the tube with water-soluble lubricant.

> **Never lubricate an NG tube with a lubricant such as petroleum jelly. The patient may aspirate and develop lipoid pneumonia.**

5 Put on gloves. Now you're ready to begin insertion. Ask the patient to hold her head upright in a normal position. As shown, steady the patient's head with one hand, hold the catheter near the lower end, and insert the tube in the nostril you selected earlier. Following the tube's natural curve, gently advance it along the floor of the nasal passage.

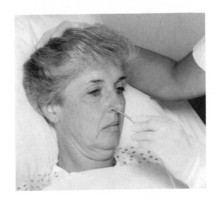

To make insertion easier, direct the tube toward the patient's ear on that side, not her other nostril. As the tip approaches her nasopharynx, rotate the tube 180 degrees inward, toward the other nostril. Continue to advance it gently until it's in the nasopharynx, pointing toward the esophagus.

> **Work slowly. If you feel resistance at any point, stop at once and withdraw the tube. Then, relubricate it and try the other nostril.**

As the tubing enters the patient's nasopharynx, she may gag. To prevent vomiting, stop advancing the tube and tell the patient to take several deep breaths or ask her to swallow water through a straw. Either action will relax the pharynx and calm the gag reflex. In addition, the water will lubricate the tube.

Allow the patient a short rest. If she continues to gag, examine her throat. The tubing may be coiled there. If it is, withdraw it until it's straight.

6 When the patient's calm again, ask her to drop her head so her chin rests on her chest. This position will close her trachea and open her esophagus. Slowly advance the tubing into the esophagus.

If the patient continues to gag, ask her to sip water while you advance the tube all the way to her stomach. Or ask her to chew ice chips throughout the procedure. Advance the tubing 3" to 5" (7.6 to 12.7 cm) each time she swallows.

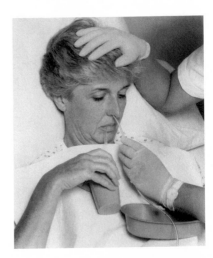

COMPARING GASTRIC TUBES

DESCRIPTION	ADVANTAGE	DISADVANTAGE
Dubbhoff tube: small bore, very flexible, stylet used during insertion	Easy insertion with minimal trauma into the stomach or duodenum	Small diameter increases risk of obstruction. Confirming placement may require X-ray.
Ewald tube: rubber, large gauge, unvented	Insertion through the mouth, usually for lavage	Persons who are unfamiliar with the tube may attempt nasal insertion.
Levin tube: rubber or plastic single lumen, unvented	Simple, commonly used	Use with suction can cause adherence to gastric mucosa and lead to injury or obstruction.
Salem sump: plastic, double lumen, vented	Vented to prevent adherence to gastric mucosa	Vent must be kept patent and not be used for irrigation.

NURSING TIP If the patient isn't permitted water or ice chips, ask her to swallow at your signal.

Continue the process until you have inserted the tube to the correct length. If you can't insert it that far, the tube may be in the patient's trachea, not her esophagus. Other signs that the tube may be in her trachea are vapor in the tubing and respiratory distress. Withdraw the tubing at once.

7 Even if the patient shows no sign of respiratory distress, make sure the tube is in her stomach, not a lung, before you proceed. To verify placement, first attempt to aspirate gastric fluid with a bulb or a piston syringe as shown. You should be able to aspirate fluid easily, unless the tube is pressed against the stomach wall. If you have trouble, withdraw the tube slightly and try again. If you still can't aspirate gastric fluid, the tube is probably in a lung.

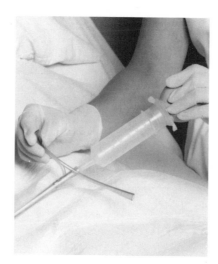

If you have successfully aspirated stomach contents, flush the tube with 30 ml normal saline solution to clear gastric fluid from the tube. Next, place a stethoscope over the patient's stomach, attach the syringe to the tube, and inject about 15 cc of air. If you hear a swooshing sound, air has entered her stomach. Silence usually indicates that the air's been absorbed by lung tissue.

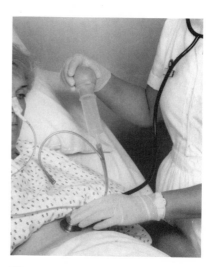

8 Before taping, make sure the bridge of the nose is clean and dry. Apply skin adhesive to the bridge of the nose.

Cut or tear an appropriate size of adhesive tape for the length of the patient's nose, about 3" to 4" (7.6 to 10.2 cm). Then, cut or tear half of the tape in half lengthwise and apply tape to bridge of nose.

9 Loop the torn pieces of tape around the tube below the nostrils as shown. Tape tube to the face or loop the tape over ear to move it away from the patient's face.

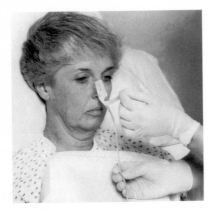

Commercial products are available that secure the NG tube and cushion the nose as well.

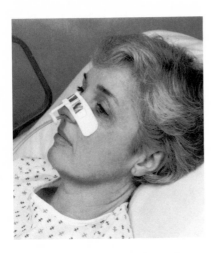

After taping, plug or clamp the end of the tubing. Cover the open end of the tube with gauze to keep it clean. (If using a Salem sump tube, cap the tube by fitting the blue pigtail over the 5-in-1 adapter)

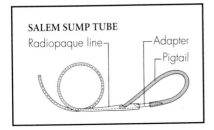

SALEM SUMP TUBE
Radiopaque line—
—Adapter
—Pigtail

However, if the patient complains of nausea, leave the tube unclamped until the nausea subsides. This provides an opening for vomitus.

10 To prevent the tube from dragging downward, wrap another piece of adhesive tape around the end of it and leave a tab. Then, safety-pin the tape tab to the patient's gown, just below shoulder level. Or, loop a rubber band around the tubing in slip-not fashion. Then, pin the rubber band to the patient's gown.

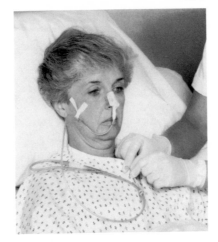

Finally, document the entire procedure. Then, to make your patient as comfortable as possible, provide good mouth and nose care. Encourage her to brush her teeth regularly.

Minimize nasal irritation by placing a small amount of water-soluble lubricant in each nostril. To prevent pressure ulcers, check the patient regularly to make sure the tubing is positioned comfortably.

How to give medication through an NG tube

Before you begin, double-check the medication order, using the seven "rights" system, and review any special considerations for the medication. For example, should you give it with tube feedings? If so, should you

avoid giving certain foods at the same time? The action of oral medication doesn't change just because you're using an NG tube. Make sure you know all the answers before you proceed. Then, follow these steps:

1 Measure the medication, and let it warm to room temperature. Remember, all medication given through an NG tube must be in liquid form. Do not dilute liquid medication. Then, gather the following equipment: bulb syringe, normal saline solution, tissues, gloves, bed-saver pads, clamp, emesis basin, and stethoscope. If you prefer not to use a bulb syringe, substitute a small funnel or a 50-ml piston syringe. (Never use a syringe smaller than 20 ml.)

2 After checking the medication order again, help the patient sit up. Remove the clamp or plug from the NG tube as shown. Then, confirm that the tube is placed in her stomach using the techniques discussed on page 21. Protect the patient's gown with a bedsaver pad or a towel, and offer tissues, in case she salivates excessively during the procedure. Put on gloves. Next, clamp the tube with a hemostat or by pinching it between your fingers.

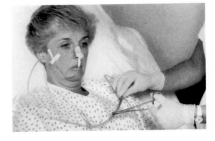

3 Remove the bulb or piston from the syringe (unless you're using a funnel), and attach the syringe to the tube.

As shown, pour the medication into the syringe. Unclamp or release the tubing, and let the medication flow through it by gravity. Never force liquids down an NG tube.

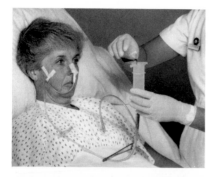

> **Throughout the procedure, watch the patient's reactions. Stop immediately if she shows signs of discomfort. To control the flow of liquid, raise or lower the syringe height, or pinch and release the tube.**

Before the syringe empties completely, begin flushing the tube with 30 to 50 ml water. (For a child, use only 20 to 25 ml of water.)

If you don't flush the tube, much of the medication will remain on the tube's sides and will never reach the patient. Flushing also clears medication from the openings at the end of the tube, and reduces the chance of clogging.

4 After you've administered all the medication and water, remove the syringe or funnel, and clamp or plug the tube. If the patient complains of nausea, leave the tube open until the feeling subsides.

Then, ask the patient to remain sitting in bed for approximately 30 minutes.

If she's uncomfortable sitting, position her on her right side, with the head of the bed partially elevated

as shown. Either position will encourage her stomach to empty and will discourage regurgitation.

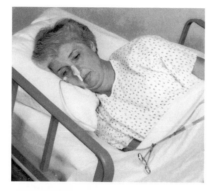

NURSING TIP   A few medications, such as antacids, should stay in the patient's stomach longer. To discourage gastric emptying after administering such drugs, position the patient on her left side, with the head of the bed slightly elevated, and clamp the NG tube for 30 minutes, or as ordered.

5 Document the entire procedure.

How to remove an NG tube

1 Ask the patient to sit upright, or place her in a high Fowler's position. Protect her gown with a towel or bedsaver pad. Release the tube that's pinned to her gown, and untape it from her nose.

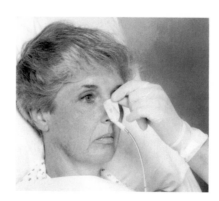

Now, gently rotate the tube to make sure it moves freely. If it doesn't, try flushing the tube with 30 ml normal saline solution and gravity. If the tube still won't move freely, notify the doctor.

2 After you've checked the tube, get ready to withdraw it. Ask the patient to take and hold a deep breath. Reclamp the NG tube with a hemostat, or fold it in your hand, as shown. This will prevent any fluid in the tube from running down the patient's throat and getting into her lungs during withdrawal.

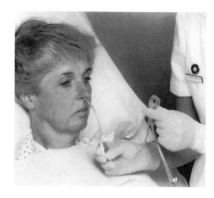

Then slowly withdraw the tube onto a towel out of the patient's sight, if possible. When you're finished, tell the patient to resume normal breathing.

Finally, document the entire procedure.

How to give medication through a gastrostomy tube

A gastrostomy tube is an indwelling (Foley) catheter or other tube that has been surgically inserted into the stomach through the abdominal wall to feed the patient. It can also be used to administer medication as follows.

1 Gather the following equipment: bulb syringe, liquid medication,

60 ml water or irrigant, bedsaver pad, 4" × 4" sterile gauze pads, rubber band, 2" (5.1 cm) tape, emesis basin, and gloves. (If you prefer, use a funnel instead of a syringe.) Make sure the medication is in liquid form and at room temperature.

2 After you've double-checked the order using the seven "rights" system, help the patient to a sitting or high Fowler's position. Put on gloves. Protect the bed with a towel or bedsaver pad, and expose the gastrostomy site.

Uncap the tube or unclamp it. Test the tube for patency by aspirating gastric contents. Instill 30 ml of the irrigant into the tube, but don't pour all the solution in at once. Instead, make sure the flow into the tube is slow and steady. If the liquid backs up, suspect a nonpatent tube. Try to free it by gently twisting it between your fingers.

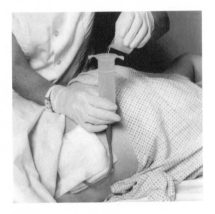

3 Pour medication into the syringe. Make sure it flows slowly and steadily through the gastrostomy tube.

If you feel resistance, or the medication leaks from around the gastrostomy tube, stop the procedure and flush the tube again. If unsuccessful, stop the procedure and notify the doctor.

Follow the medication with at least 30 ml water to clear the tube.

Remove the syringe, and replace the tube's cap or clamp.

3 Wrap a 4" × 4" sterile gauze pad around the tube's open end to keep it clean. Then, secure the gauze with a rubber band, as shown.

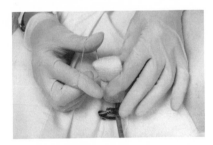

Now, examine the patient's gastrostomy site. Has any gastric drainage spilled onto his abdomen? If so, wash the area with water or saline and dry it thoroughly. Redress the site if necessary.

How to irrigate a nonpatent gastrostomy tube

1 If the tube isn't sutured in place internally or externally, gently twist it between your fingers, as shown. If the tube is sutured in place, try repositioning the patient. For example, elevate his head, or turn the patient on his left side. If the tube's tip is pressed against the stomach wall, these movements may free it.

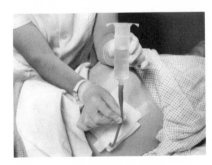

2 If that doesn't work, compress the bulb and attach it to the syringe. Then, withdraw the water from the

gastric tube. Remove the syringe and expel the water into a container. Then, reattach the syringe to the tube and try aspirating stomach contents.

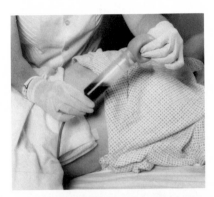

> **Never aspirate forcefully. If the tip of the tube is pressed against the stomach wall, vigorous aspiration may injure the gastric mucosa.**

3 If this method doesn't work, add 30 ml of water to the syringe. Compress the bulb firmly to push the fluid through the tube. Then, gently withdraw the fluid.

If you still have difficulty, use the syringe to inject 20 cc of air into the tube. Then, try aspirating again. The gastrostomy tube may need to be replaced. Check the stoma site and then, if ordered, replace the tube following institution policy.

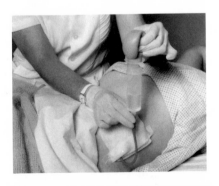

NURSING CONSIDERATIONS: GASTROSTOMY TUBES

- Before administering medication into the tube, assess skin for irritation caused by gastric secretions. Change dressings if necessary.
- Change tubing, enteral feeding bags, and pump administration sets daily or as frequently as institution policy requires.
- Check patency of the tube regularly, every 2 to 4 hours or as policy requires.
- Flush the tube with 30 ml of fluid after every intermittent feeding or drug instillation.
- If the tube is used for continuous feeding, flush it every shift and after every drug instillation.
- Fluids that can be used to flush tubes include normal saline, water, cranberry juice, or carbonated beverages. The preferred fluid is water, which is most effective in flushing clogged tubes.
- To prevent instillation of too much fluid (more than 400 ml at one time for an adult), schedule drug instillation so it does not coincide with the patient's tube feeding. If both must be scheduled simultaneously, give the medication first to ensure that the patient receives the prescribed drug therapy even if he cannot tolerate an entire feeding. However, check to avoid a drug and food interaction or incompatibility.
- Give liquid medications only. Avoid oily preparations because they cling to the sides of the tube and resist mixing with the irrigating solution. Crushing enteric or sustained-release tablets destroys their intended effect and occludes the feeding tube.
- If the patient is receiving medications such as antacids that should remain in the stomach longer, position him on his left side with the head of the bed slightly elevated to discourage gastric emptying. Clamp the tube or hold feeding for 30 minutes.
- Be aware of the osmolality of certain drugs. Hyperosmolar drugs such as potassium chloride elixir cause diarrhea. Notify the dietitian and pharmacist about the need to adjust feeding components.
- Know that certain drugs such as phenytoin (Dilantin) and theophylline (Slo-phyllin) bind with tube feedings. Schedule administration of these drugs at times when a continuous feeding can be stopped or before intermittent feedings. Stop continuous feedings 1 hour before drug administration.

How to change a gastrostomy dressing

Obtain some precut drainage sponges or make them yourself by holding two wrapped 4" × 4" gauze pads together and cutting a slit halfway through the middle. Commercially available skin barriers are another option. Consider product availability, cost, patient preference, and skin condition when making your selection.

Place the patient in the supine position and expose the abdomen. Put on gloves. Next, clean the area around the gastrostomy site with warm water (gastrostomy tubes don't fit snugly, so irritating acidic secretions or feeding solution may leak around the tube and cause skin excoriation).

Using drainage sponge dressings

1 If the tube isn't held firmly in place by sutures, tape it to the patient's abdomen chevron style.

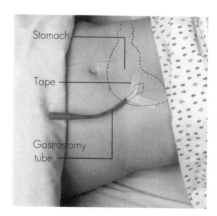

2 Take the two 4" × 4" gauze pads out of their wrappers, and fit them snugly around the tube so the slit sides overlap.

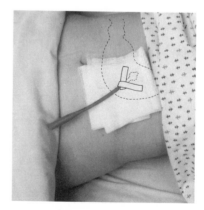

Now, place an uncut 4" × 4" gauze pad directly on top of the two slit pads. Secure it with two strips of 2" (5.1 cm) tape.

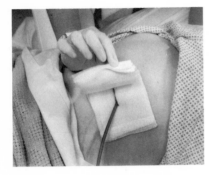

Using adhesive skin wafer dressings

1 Apply skin adhesive to area surrounding site (except when skin is excoriated).

2 Enlarge the center hole on the skin wafer (Stomahesive) to a size that will encircle the feeding tube.

3 Release the paper backing on the wafer and place the wafer hole over the distal end of the gastrostomy tube and slide it down to the abdomen. Press the wafer onto the patient's skin.

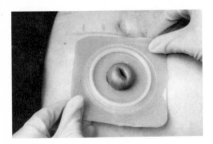

4 Secure the gastrostomy tube to the wafer with tape (chevron style). Place a dry sterile dressing directly over the wafer.

Teaching gastrostomy care

As soon as your patient is able to care for his gastrostomy, show him how. But remember, he'll probably need some extra support from you. Most likely, he'll have a hard time accepting the change in his body image and the loss of normal eating habits. You can help hasten the adjustment by giving the patient some control over his own care.

When you administer food or medication or change the dressing, explain the procedure in words he can understand. Begin by having the patient perform simple tasks to increase his confidence. For example, start by encouraging him to help with removal of sterile dressings. Encourage him to ask questions. Then, make sure you're nearby the first few times he tries each procedure himself in case he needs help or encouragement.

How to reinsert a gastrostomy tube with an indwelling catheter

After you have verified the doctor's order to replace the gastrostomy tube and determined that the site is well healed, identify the size and type of tube in place. Gather the following equipment: indwelling (Foley) catheter (the same size as currently being used), water soluble lubricant, 10-ml syringe, 20- or 50-ml syringe, emesis basin, sterile water, adhesive skin wafer or sterile gauze pads, 2" (5.1 cm) tape, gloves, and bedsaver pad.

Provide privacy and explain the procedure. Reassure the patient that it will not be painful.

1 Assist the patient into a supine position to expose the abdomen. Place a bedsaver pad under the patient. Put on gloves. Inspect the stoma for color and the skin for excoriation.

2 Gently remove all dressings and deflate the catheter baloon by withdrawing the water. Carefully pull the catheter free from the site.

3 Place water-soluble lubricant on the clean catheter tip and insert it into the stomach opening about 1" (2.5 cm) beyond the balloon. Inflate the balloon with 2 to 4 ml of sterile water using a 10-ml syringe.

Apply gentle pressure to the catheter and tape it in place (see How to Change a Gastrostomy Dressing).

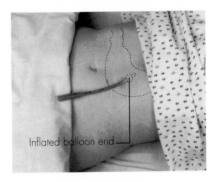

Inflated balloon end

4 Aspirate for stomach contents to verify tube placement in the stomach. Test the aspirate with a reagent strip to confirm acid pH.

5 Assist the patient to a comfortable position and document the procedure.

The button device: An alternative to the gastrostomy tube

The gastrostomy feeding button (The Button), a commercially available device, functions like a gastrostomy tube by delivering enteral feedings and medications directly into the stomach. However, this device, which fits flush to the patient's skin, requires no dressing and is cosmetically more acceptable to the patient.

How to use a gastrostomy button for enteral feeding

The patient's doctor will prescribe the enteral feeding. This order should include the type of feeding (bolus or continuous), the formula to be instilled, the flow rate, and the amount of water to be administered after each feeding. Occasionally, the doctor may want you to decompress (release accumulated air) the stomach either before or after a feeding.

To decompress the stomach of a patient with a button device, simply inactivate the antireflux valve by passing the appropriately sized decompression tube, shown here, through the valve. Then, allow the stomach to deflate for the prescribed amount of time.

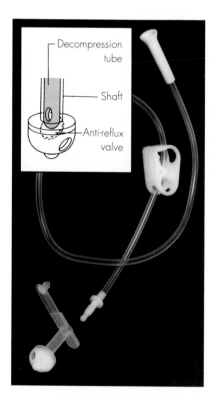

Assemble the following equipment: gloves, feeding tubing, 10-ml syringe, and formula. Then proceed as follows:

1 Assist the patient into an upright position.

2 Put on gloves and open the safety plug on top of the device.

3 Attach the feeding tubing set to the device, as shown.

4 To ensure that the device is patent, draw up 5 to 10 ml of water (3 to 5 ml for children) into a syringe and, after inserting the syringe into the device, inject the water. If the water won't go in, try repositioning the patient. If the water still won't go in, notify the doctor. *Do not begin the feeding.*

5 If you have verified patency, attach the feeding container to the tubing.

6 Open the feeding tube clamp and adjust the flow to the prescribed rate.

7 Add the prescribed amount of water to the feeding container *before* all of the formula has been instilled so air doesn't accidentally enter the stomach, creating gas and causing discomfort.

How to use the gastrostomy button to give medication

If medication is prescribed for the patient with a button device, ask the doctor to order the liquid form if possible; if not, you may administer a tablet or capsule if it is dissolved in 30 to 50 ml (15 to 30 ml for children) of warm water. To administer medication this way, follow steps 1, 2, and 3 of the feeding procedure, and then proceed as follows:

4 Draw the medication into a syringe and inject it into the feeding tubing.

5 Withdraw the medication syringe and flush the tubing with 50 ml (30 ml for children) of warm water. Now, replace the safety plug.

6 Keep the patient upright at a 30-degree angle for 30 minutes after giving the medication.

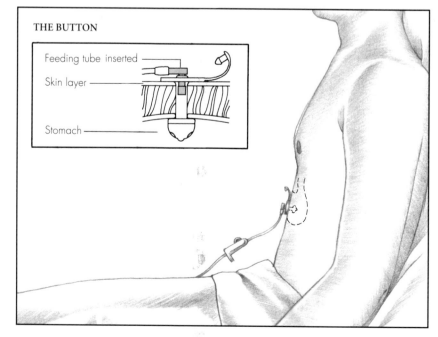

THE BUTTON

Feeding tube inserted

Skin layer

Stomach

NURSING CONSIDERATIONS: GASTROSTOMY BUTTON

The following nursing tips will help you maintain button patency and prevent discomfort or complications.

• There is no need to keep a dressing over a button device, but daily cleaning around the device with mild soap and water is necessary. Because patients with a button device are allowed to bathe, this is a good time to clean the device.

• Rotate the button device once daily.

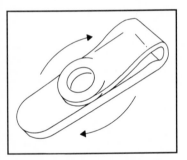

• Instruct the patient to check the site for redness, pain or soreness, swelling, or unusual drainage. Report any of these signs to the doctor. (Swelling of the stoma may indicate that the patient has outgrown the existing device and needs a larger one.)

• Always allow the site to air dry thoroughly before covering it with clothing.

• Flush the device with water before and after feedings and drug instillation. (The interior may be gently cleaned with a cotton-tipped applicator if residue build-up if suspected.)

• If the patient complains of fullness, the antireflux valve may be stuck in the open position. To check the valve, insert the decompression tube into the button shaft. If you hear a click or feel the valve close, you may have corrected the problem. However, if the patient's discomfort persists, notify the doctor.

• Observe for leakage around the tube, which may indicate a malfunctioning antireflux valve, inappropriate button size, or the need for stomach decompression.

Rectal Administration

Using the rectal route for systemic effects

The doctor may want you to give your patient medication by the rectal route because of these advantages:
• It provides a safe route for the patient who is vomiting, unconscious, or unable to swallow.
• It provides an effective route to treat vomiting.
• It doesn't irritate the patient's upper GI tract, as some oral medications do.
• It avoids destruction of medication by digestive enzymes in the stomach and small intestine.
• It avoids biotransformation in the liver because drugs absorbed from the lower rectum bypass the portal system.

However, the rectal route also has these disadvantages:
• It may be uncomfortable and embarrassing for the patient.
• It may result in irregular or incomplete drug absorption, depending on the patient's ability to retain the medication and on the presence of feces in his rectum. Because rectal absorption may be incomplete, rectal dosages of some medications may be larger than oral doses.
• It may stimulate the patient's vagal nerve by stretching his anal sphincters. For this reason, you must use the rectal route cautiously with cardiac patients.

Don't administer a laxative to a patient with undiagnosed abdominal pain. If the pain is a symptom of appendicitis, increased peristaltic action could rupture the appendix.

How to apply rectal ointments

The patient whose rectum is sore or inflamed may need application of a rectal ointment for its soothing, local effect. To apply it internally, use a rectal applicator placed on the end of the tube.

1 Get the prescribed tube of ointment and a tapered applicator with openings along the sides. Also obtain water-soluble lubricant, a bedsaver pad, several 4" × 4" gauze pads, and gloves.

2 Provide privacy for your patient and explain what you're going to do. Then position the patient on her side with her top leg flexed, so you can see her anus easily. (If she can't tolerate a side position, you may substitute one that's more comfortable.) Protect the bedding with a bedsaver pad. Put on gloves.

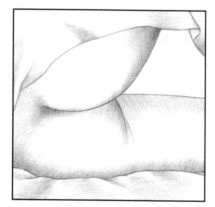

3 Expect to use approximately 1" (2.5 cm) of ointment. To gauge how much pressure to use, try squeezing out the correct amount before you attach the tube to the applicator, and coat the applicator with water-soluble lubricant.

Expose the patient's anus with one hand, and ask the patient to take sev-

eral deep breaths through her mouth, to relax her anal sphincters.

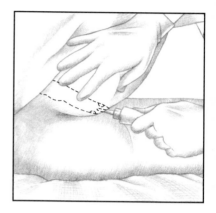

Then, slowly insert the applicator into the patient's anus, directing it toward her umbilicus. Keep in mind that the patient's rectum is probably tender, so be gentle.

When you've inserted the entire applicator, slowly squeeze the tube to eject the medication. Remove the applicator.

4 Place a folded 4" × 4" gauze pad between the patient's buttocks to absorb excess ointment. Disassemble the tube and applicator, and recap the tube. Clean the applicator thoroughly with warm water and soap. Finally, document the procedure.

How to insert a suppository

1 Wash your hands and gather the equipment you'll need: the suppository, gloves, and water-soluble lubricant. If the suppository's too soft, it will stick to the wrapper. Remedy this by holding the closed package under cold running water until it becomes firm or placing the package in the medication refrigerator for several minutes.

GUIDE TO RECTAL MEDICATIONS

DESCRIPTION	LOCAL USE	SYSTEMIC USE
Suppository		
A solid medication in a firm base, such as cocoa butter, that melts at body temperature. May be molded in a variety of cylindrical shapes. Usually abut 1 1/2" (4 cm) long (smaller for infants and children). Keep refrigerated before use to maintain firmness.	• Analgesics • Astringents • Antipruritics • Anti-inflammatory agents • Laxatives, lubricants, and cathartics • Carminatives	• Analgesics • Antiemetics • Antipyretics • Bronchodilators • Sedatives • Hypnotics
Enema		
Liquid given as either a retention enema (retained by the patient for at least 30 minutes or until absorbed) or a nonretention enema (retained by the patient for at least 10 minutes and then expelled). *Note:* Enemas given to clean the lower bowel aren't medicated.	• Anthelmintics • Astringents • Laxatives, lubricants, and cathartics • Antiseptics • Steroids	• Antipyretics • Sedatives • Anesthetics • Nutritives and water
Ointment		
A semisolid medication that may be applied externally to the anus or internally to the rectum.	• Antipruritics • Astringents • Analgesics and anesthetics • Anti-inflammatory agents • Antiseptics	• None

2 Provide privacy for your patient by closing her door and drawing the bed curtains. Explain the procedure, and position her so her anus is exposed. (Choose any position that she finds comfortable.)

> **Is the patient unconscious? Don't let this keep you from explaining the procedure. Remember, an unconscious patient may later recall everything you said. Your reassuring words will encourage her to relax.**

3 Put on a glove. Remove the suppository from the wrapper, and lubricate it with water-soluble lubricant.

With your ungloved hand, separate the patient's buttocks so you can see her anus. Ask her to take a deep breath. With your gloved hand, gently insert the suppository into her rectum, tapered end first. Use your forefinger to direct it along the rectal wall toward the umbilicus. Continue to advance it 3" (7.6 cm), or about the length of your finger, until it's passed the patient's internal anal sphincter (see inset). Otherwise, it may be expelled.

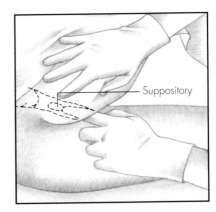

Suppository

> **Take care not to push the suppository into a fecal mass.**

4 When the suppository is in place, hold the patient's buttocks together or press on her anus with a 4" × 4" gauze pad or tissues until her urge to defecate subsides. Then, clean excess lubricant from the anus.

5 Urge the patient to retain the suppository for at least 20 minutes. Advise her that the suppository may discolor her next bowel movement. Bismuth subgallate (Anusol) suppositories, for example, give feces a silver-gray, pasty appearance. Remove your glove or finger cot, wash your hands, and document the procedure.

How to administer a nonretention enema

1 Obtain a disposable enema kit. You'll also need the following equipment: an I.V. pole, an enema bag or can, solution and tubing, slide clamp, bedsaver pad, water-soluble lubricant, paper towel, 4" × 4" gauze pad, a bedpan, and gloves.

Heat the solution to between 100° and 105° F (40.7° to 40.6° C). Pour the warmed solution into the enema container and hang the container 12" to 18" (37.8 to 46 cm) above the bed. If a female patient has a condition affecting her reproductive organs, hang the container level with her upper hip.

2 Close the door and the bed curtain to ensure privacy. Explain the procedure and position the patient on her left side with the top leg flexed so the anus is visible. Put on gloves, flush tubing or compress container, if using a bag, to clear out air. Clamp the tubing. Place a bedsaver pad under the patient's buttocks.

NURSING CONSIDERATIONS: SUPPOSITORIES

If you gave the suppository to relieve constipation, tell your patient to defecate as soon as she feels an urge.

Because intake of food and fluid stimulates peristalsis, insert a suppository to relieve constipation about 30 minutes before mealtime to help soften the feces in the rectum and facilitate defecation.

3 Lubricate the tip of the tubing, further expose the patient's anus and ask her to breathe deeply. Gently insert the tube about 3" to 4" (7.6 to 10.2 cm) into the rectum. Open the tubing clamp slightly and allow the solution to flow slowly. If the patient experiences cramping or pain, ask her to take a deep breath while you pinch the tubing to reduce the flow until the sensation passes. When the solution has been instilled, clamp the tubing and remove the tube gently.

NOTE Don't let the container become completely empty before you clamp it or you may introduce air into the rectum.

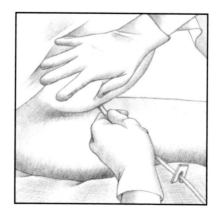

4 Pressing on the patient's anus with a 4" × 4" gauze pad may help subdue the urge to defecate. Keep the bedpan within the patient's reach but encourage her to retain the enema for at least 10 minutes before expelling it.

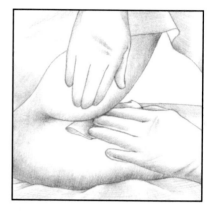

5 Once the enema has been expelled, wash and dry the patient's anal area, and return her to a comfortable position. Ventilate her room, using an air freshener if necessary. Document the procedure, including the type and amount of solution used, color and consistency of expelled feces, amount of flatus expelled, reduction in abdominal distension, if any, and patient's tolerance of the procedure.

How to administer a prepackaged enema

Commercially prepared hypertonic enemas are usually small, prepackaged, rapid-acting instillations. The most commonly used is the sodium biphosphate-sodium phosphate (Fleet) enema, which administers only a small amount of fluid (approximately 120 ml). This enema should not be used in small children because the hypertonic solution causes a shift of fluid from the circulatory system and subcutaneous tissue that can result in hypovolemia.

1 Assemble the following equipment: prepackaged enema, bedsaver pad, 4" × 4" gauze pad, bed pan, and gloves. Close the door to the room. Wash your hands and put on gloves. Bring the prepared enema to the bedside. Draw the curtains around the bed. Explain the procedure, place a bedsaver pad under the patient and assist her into a left Sims' position.

2 Squeeze the container gently to expel air. Separate the buttocks to further expose the anus. Instruct the patient to take a deep breath; simultaneously insert the nozzle into the anus, pointing toward the umbilicus. Continue to squeeze the container until you have instilled all of the solution.

Complete and document the procedure (see How to Administer a Nonretention Enema).

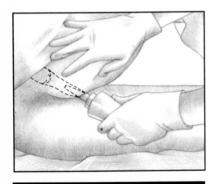

Preparing to give a medicated retention enema

Giving a medicated retention enema requires good planning. For example, you must schedule the procedure before meals because a full stomach triggers peristalsis, which makes retention difficult.

Before beginning the procedure, carefully check your patient's condition. Notify the doctor if:
• the patient is constipated. Feces in the rectum will interfere with drug absorption. The doctor may order a cleansing nonretention enema first.

• the patient has diarrhea. In this case, the drug may be expelled before it can be absorbed. The doctor may want you to check for a fecal impaction before he treats the diarrhea. Then, he may want to choose another route.
• the patient has an inflamed rectum. An enema may exacerbate the condition. The doctor may want to choose another route.

Always take enough time to thoroughly prepare the patient for this procedure. Because you'll need the patient's cooperation, make sure he understands its purpose and the importance of retaining the medication until it's absorbed. Finally, to reduce the risk of stimulating peristalsis during the procedure, ask the patient to empty his bladder and rectum before you begin.

How to administer a retention enema

1 Gather the equipment shown: a pitcher or other small container to hold the enema solution, a bulb syringe (with bulb removed), a rectal tube or catheter, water-soluble lubricant, a bedsaver pad, a paper towel, 4" × 4" gauze pads or tissues, a bedpan, a hemostat, and gloves.

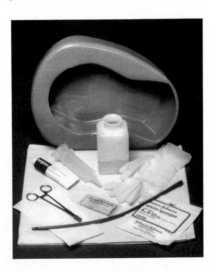

To avoid stimulating peristalsis when you give the enema, heat the solution to between 100° and 105° F (37.8° and 40.6° C) before administering it. To confirm the temperature, test it with a bath thermometer or pour a little of the solution over the inside of your wrist.

2 Provide privacy by closing the door and pulling the bed curtain. Assess your patient's condition, and explain the procedure. Put on gloves. Adjust the bed so it's flat. Then, position your patient on her left side, with her right knee flexed. This will permit the enema solution to flow naturally into the descending colon.

If this position is uncomfortable for your patient, place her on her right side or back instead.

To protect the bed linen, place the bedsaver pad under the patient's left buttock. Tuck part of the pad between her legs, as shown, to catch any leakage of fluid from her rectum. Expose her anus, but provide a drape so she has some privacy. Reassure her so she won't be unduly embarrassed.

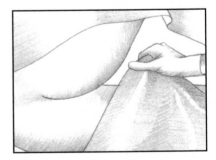

3 Flush air from the tube. To do this, first remove the bulb from the syringe, and attach the syringe to the tube. Next, double up the tube in one hand, and pour in a small amount of solution. Then, lower the open end of the tube. When the solution flows out the end, pinch the tube between your fingers, as shown.

GUIDE TO ENEMAS

Use this chart as a guide when you give a patient an enema. But before you decide which guidelines are appropriate, consider the medication the doctor has prescribed, as well as the patient's age, size, and condition. For instance, if the patient's a small 9-year-old child, use the smallest tube suggested for his age-group. Physical size is more important than age.

Always use smaller tubing and less solution when you give a retention enema. This combination will create less pressure in the patient's rectum and make retention easier.

NOTE: Never give a retention enema to an infant or young child. Neither will be able to retain it.

AGE-GROUP	RECTAL TUBE SIZE	LENGTH OF TUBE TO INSERT	VOLUME OF FLUID TO INTRODUCE
Retention enemas			
Adults	#14 to #20 French	3" to 4" (7.6 to 10.1 cm)	150 to 200 ml
Children over age 6	#12 to #14 French	2" to 3" (5.1 to 7.6 cm)	75 to 150 ml
Nonretention enemas			
Adults	#22 to #30 French	3" to 4" (7.6 to 10.1 cm)	750 to 1,000 ml
Children over age 6	#14 to #18 French	2" to 3" (5.1 to 7.6 cm)	500 to 1,000 ml
Children over age 2	#12 to #14 French	1 1/2" to 2" (3.8 to 5.1 cm)	500 ml or less
Infants	#12 French	1" to 1 1/2" (2.5 to 3.8 cm)	250 ml or less

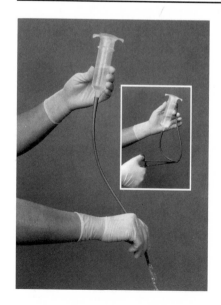

Once again, fold the tube in one hand. Then clamp it, as shown in the inset. Leave the syringe attached.

4 Place a little water-soluble lubricant on a paper towel. Lubricate the tip of the tube by rolling it in the lubricant.

With your free hand, separate the patient's buttocks, so you can see her anus. Ask the patient to breathe deeply through her mouth to help relax her anal sphincters. With your other hand, gently insert the tube, and direct it toward the patient's umbilicus.

Advance the tube about 4" (10.2 cm). Make sure it's past the internal anal sphincters or it may be expelled.

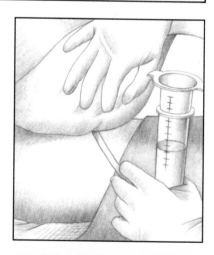

If you feel any resistance, withdraw the tube and notify the doctor. Forcing it may damage the patient's mucous membranes.

NURSING CONSIDERATIONS: ENEMAS

• Because patients with salt-retention disorders, such as congestive heart failure, may absorb sodium from a saline enema solution, administer these to such patients with caution and monitor electrolyte status.

• Schedule a retention enema before meals, because a full stomach may stimulate peristalsis and make retention difficult.

• An oil retention enema is frequently followed 1 hour later by a soap-and-water enema to help expel softened feces completely.

• When giving a hypertonic enema, use less solution because osmotic pull moves fluid into the colon from body tissues, increasing fluid volume within the colon.

• Alternative means of instilling the solution include using a bulb syringe or a funnel with the rectal tube.

• For a patient who cannot tolerate a supine position (because of dyspnea, for example), administer the enema with the head of the bed at a 30-degree angle.

• For a bedridden patient who must use a bedpan to expel the enema, raise the head of the bed so his position approximates sitting or squatting.

• Unless absolutely necessary, do not give an enema to a patient who is in a sitting position, because the solution will not flow high enough into the colon and will only distend the rectum and trigger rapid expulsion. Attempting to insert the rectal catheter into a seated patient can also injure the rectal wall.

• If the doctor orders enemas until clear, give no more than three to avoid excessive irritation of the rectal mucosa. Advise the doctor if the return is not clear after three administrations.

• In patients with fluid and electrolyte disturbances, measure the amount of expelled solution to assess for retention of enema fluid.

• Enemas may produce dizziness or faintness; excessive irritation of the colonic mucosa, from repeated administration or from patient sensitivity to enema ingredients; hyponatremia or hypokalemia, from repeated administration of hypotonic solutions; colonic water absorption, from prolonged retention of hypotonic solutions (which may in turn cause hypervolemia or water intoxication); and cardiac arrhythmias, from vasovagal reflex stimulation after insertion of the rectal catheter.

• Sodium polystyrene sulfonate enemas should be given cautiously to a patient with low sodium tolerance.

---

5 Hold the syringe about 5" (12.7 cm) above her anus. Slowly pour the warmed solution from the container into the syringe.

Next, remove the clamp, and let the solution flow into the patient by gravity. Don't try to rush the procedure by pouring the solution faster or raising the syringe height. By increasing fluid pressure in the rectum, either action could stimulate the urge to defecate.

After administering all of the enema solution, clamp the tubing and ask the patient to take a deep breath. Then, withdraw the tube gently but quickly.

Hold the patient's buttocks together until the urge to defecate

Throughout the procedure, do your best to keep your patient comfortable. If she has cramps or an urge to defecate, stop administering the enema immediately by pinching the tube. Tell the patient to breathe deeply to help her relax. When she's comfortable again, proceed cautiously. Do everything possible to help her retain the enema.

passes. Then, wash and dry her buttocks. Remove your gloves and wash your hands.

Retention time will vary according to the type of medication. As a rule, however, the patient should retain it for at least 30 minutes.

To make retention easier, keep the patient as quiet and comfortable as possible. Leave the bedsaver pad in place, to guard against seepage, and put the bedpan within reach. Don't run water within the patient's hearing.

After the prescribed length of time, tell the patient she may defecate. Then, document the procedure.

NURSING CONSIDERATIONS: SPECIAL PATIENTS

Children
Before toilet training, children cannot control their external rectal sphincter to retain enemas. Therefore, administer enemas to children in bed with a bedpan in place.

The amount of solution must be specifically prescribed for infants and toddlers under age 2. An enema tip should be inserted only 2" to 3" (5.1 to 7.6 cm) in children; only 1" (2.5 cm) in infants.

Water or commercial enemas should not be used in infants because they can cause fatal water intoxication or hypovolemia.

Elderly patients
Elderly patients with neurologic impairment may have lost sphincter control or may be incontinent. For such patients, enemas must be administered with the patient in the supine position with a bedpan in place.

Be sure to dry the skin carefully. An elderly patient's skin is easily denuded after maceration from continued exposure to moisture.

Remember that many older adults have hemorrhoids. Closely observe the rectum as you insert a well-lubricated tube to avoid painful trauma to sensitive hemorrhoidal tissue.

Topical Administration

The three major types of topical administration are inunction (drug is applied by rubbing to create friction), instillation (drug solution is used to flush mucous membrane or skin), and inhalation (drug is applied to respiratory membrane).

How to apply nitroglycerin ointment

Unlike other medications applied to the skin, nitroglycerin ointment is used for its systemic, not local, effect. You'll use nitroglycerin ointment to dilate the veins and arteries of a patient with cardiac ischemia or angina pectoris to increase blood flow to his heart. Here's how to apply nitroglycerin ointment:

1 Make sure you have recorded the patient's baseline blood pressure so you can compare it with later readings. Gather your equipment. Nitroglycerin ointment, which is prescribed in inches, comes with a rectangular piece of ruled paper that's used to apply the medication. Confirm the medication order by checking it against the patient's Kardex. Then, squeeze the prescribed amount of ointment onto the ruled paper, as shown. (Put on gloves, if desired, to help prevent absorption of the drug should you inadvertently touch it.)

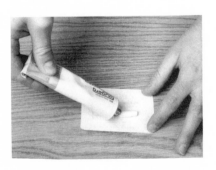

2 Tape the paper to the skin, drug side down as shown. Check institution protocol; it may require you to use the paper to apply the medication to the patient's skin (usually on the chest or arm). Spread a thin layer of the ointment over a 3" (7.6 cm) area.

3 For increased absorption, the doctor may suggest that you cover the site with plastic wrap or a transparent semipermeable dressing.

After 5 minutes, take the patient's blood pressure. If it has dropped significantly, and your patient has a headache (from vasodilation of blood vessels in his head), notify the doctor immediately. He'll probably want to decrease the next dose.

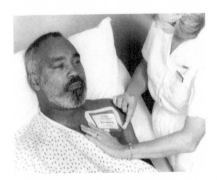

If the patient's blood pressure has dropped but he has no symptoms, instruct him to lie still until it returns to normal.

4 Document the procedure, including the time of administration, site of application, any adverse reactions (headache, postural hypotension), and the patient's overall response. If your hospital policy requires, apply a label to the site with the date, time, and your initials.

How to apply a transdermal disk

This mode of administration provides slow absorption of a drug directly into the bloodstream at a constantly controlled rate. The sustained blood level of drug with one application provides a prolonged systemic effect lasting several hours or days (a single nitroglycerin disk can provide therapeutic effect for 24 hours; a scopolamine disk for as long as 72 hours).

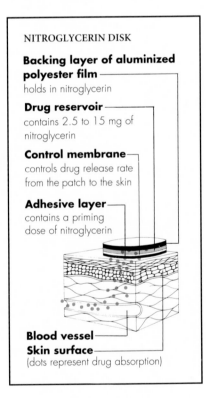

NITROGLYCERIN DISK

Backing layer of aluminized polyester film
holds in nitroglycerin

Drug reservoir
contains 2.5 to 15 mg of nitroglycerin

Control membrane
controls drug release rate from the patch to the skin

Adhesive layer
contains a priming dose of nitroglycerin

Blood vessel
Skin surface
(dots represent drug absorption)

Contraindications to application of a transdermal disk are skin allergies or reaction to the drug, open wounds or irritated skin, and calloused or scarred skin. Proceed as follows.

(Text continues on page 40.)

GUIDE TO TOPICAL DOSAGE FORMS

The chart below explains how topical dosage forms differ and how these differences affect your nursing care.

TYPE	USE	NURSING CONSIDERATIONS
Powder (inert chemical that may contain medication)	• Promotes skin drying • Reduces moisture, maceration, friction	• Apply to clean, dry skin. • To prevent inhalation of powder particles, instruct patient to turn his head to one side during application. • Before applying powder to the patient's face or neck, give him a cloth or gauze to cover his mouth. Then, ask him to exhale as you apply powder.
Lotion (suspension of insoluble powder in water or an emulsion without powder)	• Creates sensation of dryness • Leaves uniform surface film of powder • Soothes, cools, protects the skin	• Shake container well before using. • Remove residue from previous applications, if ordered. • To increase absorption in certain skin conditions, warm the patient's skin with heat packs or a bath before applying. • Apply medication to clean, dry skin. • Thoroughly massage into the skin. • After application, observe the patient's skin for local irritation.
Cream (oil-in-water emulsion in semisolid form)	• Lubricates as a barrier	• Remove residue from previous applications, if ordered. • Apply medication to clean, dry skin. • Thoroughly massage cream into the skin. • After application, observe the patient's skin for local irritation.
Ointment (a suspension of oil and water in semisolid form)	• Retains body heat • Provides prolonged medication contact	• Remove residue from previous applications, if ordered. • To increase absorption of medication, warm skin with heat packs or a bath before applying. • Apply medication to clean, dry skin. • Apply thin layer of ointment to patient's skin, and rub it in well. • Use care when applying ointment to draining wounds.
Paste (a stiff mixture of powder and ointment)	• Provides a uniform coating • Reduces and repels moisture	• Remove residue from previous applications, if ordered. • Apply medication to clean, dry skin. • Cover medication to increase absorption and to protect the patient's clothing and bed linen (see *Selecting the right dressing,* page 39).

APPLYING MEDICATION TO THE SKIN

Aways wear gloves when applying medication to the skin and provide as much privacy for the patient as possible.

BODY PART, MEDICATION	PROCEDURE	
Scalp Medicated shampoo Example: lindane (Kwell)	Shampoo the patient's hair. After drying hair and scalp, comb to remove any tangles. Apply medication to the scalp using fingertips. Spread medication evenly starting with natural part and then every 1/2" (1.3 cm). Follow product-specific instructions. Massage medication into scalp if appropriate. Repeat as instructed.	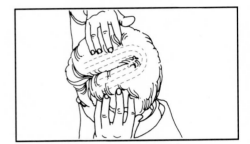
Face Topical steroid Example: betamethasone valerate (Valisone)	Wash the patient's face with mild soap and water to remove any exudate or residue. Normal saline solution, peroxide, or cottonseed or mineral oil may be used instead of soap. Apply medication to small areas (under eyes, forehead, chin) with cotton-tipped applicators, to large areas with a gauze pad. Always begin by applying medication to the patient's forehead and spread it down each side of the face to the jaw. Stroke in one direction only.	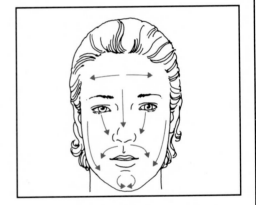
Body (trunk and extremities) Antipruritic Example: triamcinolone diacetate (Kenalog)	Examine the skin for exudate and medication residue. Clean the area, then dry it thoroughly. Use a tongue blade to remove medication from the container or squeeze small amount from tube. Remove medication from the tongue blade with a gauze pad and begin application at the midline of the neck laterally downward toward the buttocks. Follow the normal hair growth patterns. Use a clean gauze pad to remove any excess medication.	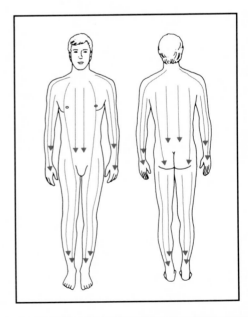

SELECTING THE RIGHT DRESSING

You'll use a medicated dressing to treat a patient's skin problems when he can't tolerate a bath, when the condition's in an area that can't be soaked, or when the condition needs long-term treatment and protection.

Dressings may be permeable, semipermeable, or occlusive. A permeable dressing allows air to reach the wound; a semipermeable dressing allows oxygen to reach the wound. An occlusive dressing is impermeable to oxygen, reduces wound pain, increases speed of re-epithelialization, and stimulates debridement and healing.

This chart explains the correct use of different types of dressings. Be sure to apply the dressing correctly. Incorrect application can macerate the site and stain clothing and linen.

TYPE	DESCRIPTION	INDICATION	EFFECTS OR BENEFITS
Open, wet dressing *(permeable)*	A dressing soaked in medication, applied to the skin, and left uncovered. When the water in the medication evaporates, the dressing is remoistened. Used, for example, to apply Burow's solution (Burosol)	• Acute inflammatory skin conditions, erosions, ulcers • Skin lesions with oozing exudate	• Delivers medication • Softens and heals the skin • Absorbs pus and exudate • Decreases blood flow to inflamed areas • Helps promote drainage
Closed, wet dressing *(occlusive)*	A dressing soaked in medication, applied to the skin, and covered with either an occlusive or insulative bandage. Covering the dressing prevents water evaporation and heat loss. An occlusive dressing is used, for example, to apply desoximetasone (Topicort); an insulative dressing, to apply boric acid solution.	• Cellulitis • Erysipelas • Psoriasis • Lichen simplex chronicus • Eczema	• Delivers medication • Softens and heals the skin • Increases effectiveness of medication • Absorbs pus and exudate • Increases blood flow to inflamed areas • Protects site from contamination
Wet to dry dressing *(permeable)*	Same as open, wet dressing, except the dressing is removed after water evaporation, not remoistened. Used, for example, to apply sodium hypochlorite (Dakin's solution).	• Wound debridement	• Delivers medication • Softens the skin • Absorbs pus, exudate, debris, eschar
Dry dressing *(semipermeable)*	An ordinary gauze pad applied to the skin. Used, for example, with debriding agent such as collagenase (Santyl).	• Neurodermatitis • Stasis dermatitis	• Protects skin from abrasion • Protects site from contamination
Transparent dressing *(semipermeable)*	Sterile filmlike dressing consisting of a thin, hypoallergenic backing and a water-resistant adhesive.	• Dressing peripheral and central I.V. catheters • Minor abrasions • Superficial pressure ulcers • Skin graft donor sites • Closed surgical wounds • Covering topical medication (unlabeled use).	• Protects site from contamination • Protects skin from abrasion • Keeps site dry • Allows visualization of site • Delivers medication (unlabeled use)

1 Verify the order on the patient's medication record and select the correct disk using the seven "rights" system.

Explain the procedure to the patient and provide privacy. Put on gloves if desired.

2 Choose a dry, hairless area (don't shave hair; clip it). The upper arm, chest, back, and the area behind the ear are the most frequently used sites. Use soap and water to clean the area where medication is to be applied.

Pull the protective backing from the disk to expose the drug. Place the disk on clean, dry skin without touching the drug, as shown.

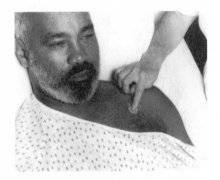

3 Wash your hands immediately to avoid absorbing the drug.

4 Document the procedure, including the time of administration, drug used, dosage, site of application, any adverse reactions (headache, postural hypotension), and the patient's response. If policy requires, apply a label to the site including the date, time, and your initials.

Mucous Membrane Administration

How to give medication by the sublingual or buccal routes

Most oral medications are swallowed and then absorbed in the lower gastrointestinal tract. But a few, such as nitroglycerin and some male hormones, may be absorbed directly into the circulation through the mucosa under the tongue (sublingual) or inside the cheek (buccal).

Systemic drug absorption via the oral mucosa offers several advantages. It permits direct entry of medication into the patient's bloodstream, so the medication takes effect quickly. In addition, it bypasses both the lower GI tract and the portal system, so the medication isn't transformed in the stomach, small intestine, or liver. And finally, the mucosal route is convenient and safe to use.

Administer sublingual and buccal tablets after all other oral medications are given. Have the patient take a swallow or two of water before giving a sublingual or buccal tablet, to stimulate saliva production and promote quicker absorption.

To give tablets via these routes, put on gloves and follow these instructions:

Sublingual route
Place tablet under the patient's tongue, as shown. Ask him to hold it in place until it's absorbed.

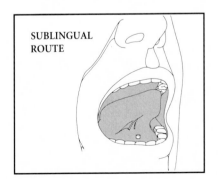

SUBLINGUAL ROUTE

Buccal route
Place tablet between the patient's cheek and teeth, as shown. Ask him to close his mouth and hold the tablet against his cheek until it's absorbed.

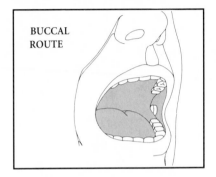

BUCCAL ROUTE

In either case, caution the patient not to swallow the tablet. Then watch him closely as the medication's being absorbed.

How to administer a translingual spray

The translingual spray also uses the mucous membranes for absorption. Nitrate preparations are available in this form and are used in patients with chronic angina.

At the onset of an anginal attack, one or two metered doses are sprayed onto the oral mucosa. The spray can also be used to prevent an anginal attack by spraying one or two doses onto the oral mucosa 5 to 10 minutes before stressful activities, such as heavy exercise, that might provoke an anginal attack.

The spray is highly flammable. Do not use it where it might be ignited.

1 The patient should be in a sitting position. Hold the canister vertically with the valve head uppermost and the spray orifice as close to the

mouth as possible. Spray the dose onto the tongue by pressing the button firmly.

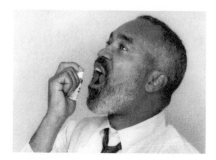

2 The patient's mouth should be closed immediately after each dose, but *the spray should not be inhaled.*

If the patient needs more than three doses within 15 minutes, notify the patient's doctor.

Instruct the patient to become familiar with the position of the spray orifice, which can be identified by the finger rest on top of the valve. Learning to handle the container easily will be particularly helpful for using the medication at night.

How to administer vaginal medication

1 Gather the following equipment: prescribed medication (suppository, cream, ointment, tablet, or gel), applicator, gloves, water-soluble lubricant, a paper towel, bedpan, bedsaver pad, several cotton balls, perineal pads, drape, and soap and water. Then, provide for the patient's privacy, and explain the procedure to her. Ask her to empty her bladder.

Insert the prescribed dose of medication into the applicator and coat the applicator tip with water or water-soluble lubricant to make insertion easier. Have the patient lie down, with her knees flexed and legs spread apart. Place a bedsaver pad under the patient to protect the bed

linen, and a drape over her legs, leaving only her perineum exposed.

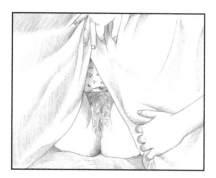

2 Put on gloves, and examine her perineum. (Know why the medication is ordered and its action. If you notice the patient's perineum is excoriated before drug administration, withhold medication and notify the doctor.) If you see any discharge, wash the area. To do this, soak several cotton balls in soapy warm water. Then, clean the left side of the perineum, the right side, and finally the center, using a fresh cotton ball for each stroke.

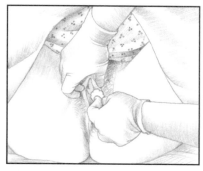

3 While the patient's labia are still separated, gently insert the applicator into her vagina. Advance the applicator about 2" (5.1 cm), angling it slightly toward her sacrum. Then, push the plunger to instill the gel, ointment, or cream, or to release the tablet or suppository, as shown. Remove the applicator and discard it, if it's disposable. If it's reusable, wash it well with warm water and soap, and return it to its container.

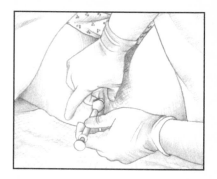

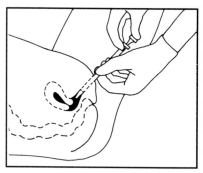

4 Tell the patient to remain lying down for about 30 minutes. If she doesn't, the medication will run out because the vagina has no sphincter. Apply perineal pads so her clothes or the bed linen don't become stained.

> **Watch her closely for possible side effects, such as increased irritation, that may be caused by the medication. Notify the doctor if any occur.**

Bladder irrigation
After bladder or prostate surgery in patients with indwelling urinary (Foley) catheters, continuous bladder irrigation may be performed to help prevent clot formation or urinary tract infection. Intermittent bladder irrigation may be performed to help maintain bladder tone. Either type of bladder irrigation uses a special triple-lumen catheter. One lumen

inflates the balloon, one directs fluid into the bladder, and one directs fluid out of the bladder.

How to administer continuous bladder irrigation

Gather the equipment needed (two containers of prescribed irrigating solution, tubing, alcohol pad, gloves, I.V. pole, bedsaver pad, and emesis basin. Provide for the patient's privacy, place the bedsaver pad under him, explain the procedure, and put on gloves.

1 Remove the protective cap from the tubing set and insert the spike

into the cleaned insertion port of the irrigation solution. Suspend the solution from the I.V. pole as shown. Squeeze the drip chamber on the spike of the tubing until it is half full.

2 Open the flow clamp until irrigation solution flows through the tubbladder distension. Then close the clamp.

3 Wipe the distal end of the tubing with an alcohol pad and insert it securely into the inflow lumen of the catheter. (The outflow lumen should already be attached to the tubing leading to the drainage collection bag.)

4 Open the flow clamp under the container of irrigating solution and set the drip rate as ordered. When the container is nearly empty, hang the second bag and repeat the procedure.

After replacing a container of solution, record the time and the

amount of fluid infused on the intake and output record. Also record the time and amount of fluid drained each time you empty the collection bag.

5 Document the time, date, appearance of drainage (cloudy, pusfilled or blood-tinged), and any complaints the patient may have. Be sure to document the administration of medicated solution on the medication Kardex.

To administer intermittent irrigation, release a clamp on the tube from the solution container and allow the specified amount of fluid to flow into the bladder. Then clamp the drainage tubing to keep the solution within the bladder for the specified period of time. After this interval, release the clamp and drain the urine and solution from the bladder. Repeat infusion followed by draining.

NURSING CONSIDERATIONS: BLADDER IRRIGATION

• When the irrigating solution contains a drug, label the container with the drug name, dose, rate, and time added.
• Always have a second container of solution available to replace the one that is nearly empty, if ordered. If none is ordered, ask the doctor to order the backup.
• Check inflow and outflow lines periodically for kinks to make sure the solution is running freely. If the flow rate is rapid, check the lines often.
• Measure outflow volume accurately. It should equal or, allowing for urine production, slightly surpass inflow volume. If inflow volume exceeds outflow volume in a patient who has had surgery, suspect bladder rupture at the suture lines or renal damage. Notify the doctor immediately.
• Empty drainage collection bags frequently, as often as every 4 hours, or as needed.

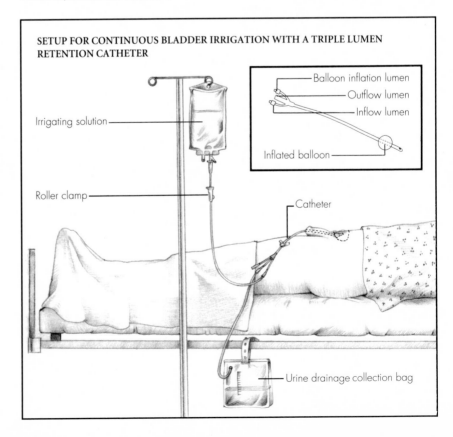

SETUP FOR CONTINUOUS BLADDER IRRIGATION WITH A TRIPLE LUMEN RETENTION CATHETER

Irrigating solution

Roller clamp

Balloon inflation lumen
Outflow lumen
Inflow lumen

Inflated balloon

Catheter

Urine drainage collection bag

How to give a sitz bath

A sitz bath is a warm water bath that is intended to increase circulation to the anal or perineal area. In most health care settings, sitz baths are given in a disposable shallow plastic basin that fits into a toilet. However, a clean bathtub may be used instead. Pain may cause the patient to be reluctant before his first sitz bath. An analgesic administered 20 minutes before may prevent or minimize discomfort.

1 Raise the toilet seat, and fit the plastic pan onto the toilet bowl. Position the pan so its drainage holes are along the back of the bowl. If you've placed the pan correctly you'll see a single slot in front.

2 Close the clamp on the bag's tubing and fill the bag with warm water and medication (if ordered).

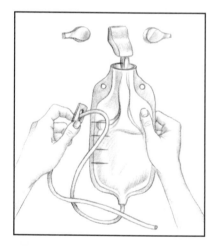

3 Snap the free end of the tubing into the slot at the front of the pan. Then, hang the bag on the door knob or towel bar. Make sure the bag's higher than the toilet

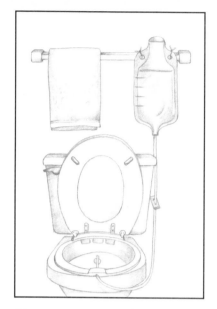

4 Provide privacy for the patient. Now, the patient is ready for the sitz bath. Assist him onto the pan, and cover the patient's shoulders and lower legs to keep him warm. Open the clamp on the tubing. Let the warm water flow from the bag and fill the pan. (Don't worry about its overflowing, because excess water will flow out the drainage holes.) The patient should sit in the pan until the water begins to cool. After the sitz bath, advise the patient to dry himself completely. If ordered by the doctor, apply an ointment or dressing.

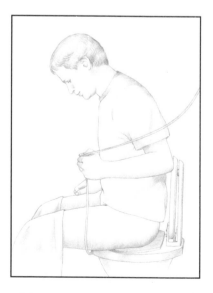

> **The patient may experience fatigue and lightheadedness at the end of the bath, especially if an analgesic is administered. Be sure to stay with the patient to ensure his saftey.**

5 Assist the patient to bed, reassess him, and document the procedure and his response to it.

Ophthalmic Administration

Medication is applied to the eye either as an ointment or as drops for therapeutic and diagnostic purposes. The administration of eye medication requires sterile technique to avoid irritation or infection. If there is visible drainage from the eyes or policy requires, wear gloves. Eye medication is usually instilled into the eye's lower conjunctival sac with resultant distribution throughout the tear film.

How to instill eye drops

1 Wash your hands thoroughly and put on gloves if necessary. Read the medication label and be sure it says "For ophthalmic use" or "For use in the eyes." Next, hold the bottle up to the light and examine it. If the medication is discolored or contains sediment, discard it immediately. However, remember that some eye suspensions are normally cloudy. If in doubt, check with the pharmacist. If the medication appears okay, warm it to room temperature by holding it between your hands for 2 minutes.

NURSING TIP Elderly patients commonly have difficulty instilling eye drops and feel unsure if the drops have gone into the eye. Chilling the eye drops before instillation allows such patients to feel correct placement of the drops.

2 Darken the patient's room if the light is irritating. With a moistened gauze pad, clean all secretions and old medication from around the patient's eye, moving from inner canthus to outer canthus. Use a fresh pad for each eye so you don't spread infection.

3 Assist the patient to a supine or sitting position.

Now, have the patient tilt his head slightly back and toward the eye you're treating. Instruct the patient to look toward the ceiling. Squeeze the bulb of the dropper to fill it with medication. With your other hand, pull down the lower eyelid to expose the conjunctiva. Then squeeze the prescribed number of drops into the exposed sac, as shown. Don't drop the medication directly onto the eyeball, and take care not to touch the dropper to the eye or eyelashes. Wipe away excess medication with a clean tissue. Repeat the procedure in the other eye, if appropriate.

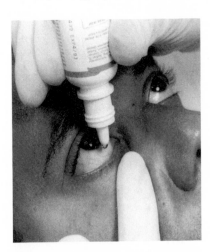

4 Discard any medication remaining in the dropper. Recap the medication and store it away from heat and light. Document the procedure and the patient's response to the drug.

NOTE When multiple eye drop prescriptions are ordered, wait at least 5 minutes between instillations to avoid excessive loss and dilution of the drugs.

How to insert and remove an eye medication disk

A medication disk inserted into the eye can release medication continuously for up to 1 week. Pilocarpine, for example, can be administered this way to treat glaucoma. The small, flexible oval disk consists of three layers: two soft outer layers and a middle layer containing the medication. Floating between the eyelids and the sclera, the disk stays in the eye while the patient sleeps and even during swimming and other athletic activities. Eye moisture or contact lenses don't adversely affect the disk. Once the disk is in place, the fluid in the eye moistens it, releasing the medication. Because eye medication disks release medication continuously, the patient never has to worry about forgetting to instill his eye drops. Contraindications to this dosage form include conjunctivitis, keratitis, retinal detachment, and any condition in which constriction of the pupil should be avoided.

Inserting an eye medication disk
Arrange to insert the disk at bedtime. This minimizes the problems caused by the blurring that occurs immediately after the disk is inserted.

1 Wash your hands and put on sterile gloves if drainage is apparent. Press your fingertip against the oval disk so its length lies horizontally across your fingertip. It should stick to your finger. Lift it out of its packet.

2 Evert the patient's lower eyelid and place the disk in the conjunctival sac. It should lie horizontally, not vertically, as shown. The disk should automatically stick to the eye.

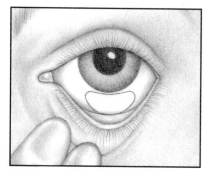

3 Pull the lower eyelid out, up, and over the disk. Tell the patient to blink several times. If the disk is still visible, lift the lower lid out and over the disk again. Tell the patient that once the disk is in place, he can adjust its position by gently pressing a finger against the closed lid. However, warn against rubbing the eye or moving the disk across the iris.

4 If the disk falls out, wash your hands, put on a new pair of gloves if necessary, rinse the disk in cool water, and reinsert it. If the disk bends out of shape, replace it with a new one. If both of the patient's eyes are being treated with medication disks, replace both disks at the same time so both eyes receive medication at the same rate.

5 If the disk continually slips out of position, reinsert the disk under the upper eyelid. To do this, gently lift and evert the upper eyelid and insert the disk in the conjunctival sac. Then, gently pull the lid back into position and tell the patient to blink several times. To adjust the disk to

the most comfortable position, have the patient gently press on the closed lid. Retaining the disk should become easier with continued use. If he can't retain it, notify the doctor.

Possible adverse reactions include foreign-body sensation in the eye, mild tearing or redness, increased mucous discharge, eyelid redness, and itchiness. Blurred vision, stinging, swelling, and headaches commonly occur with pilocarpine. Mild symptoms are common but should subside within the first 6 weeks of use.

Removing an eye medication disk
Put on gloves if necessary. You can remove an eye medication disk with one or two fingers.

1 To use one finger, evert the lower eyelid with one hand so you expose the disk. Then, use the forefinger of your other hand to slide the disk onto the lid and out of the patient's eye.

2 To use two fingers, evert the lower lid with one hand to expose the disk. Then, pinch the disk with the thumb and forefinger of your other hand and remove it from the eye.

3 If the disk is in the upper eyelid, apply long circular strokes to the patient's closed eyelid with your finger until you can see the disk in the corner of the patient's eye. When the disk is visible, place your finger directly on the disk and move it to the lower sclera. Then remove it as you would a disk in the lower lid.

How to enhance ocular drug absorption

1 To enhance drug absorption and concentration in the eye, use the pouch method of drug administra-

tion. This alternative technique uses the index finger and thumb to pull out the lower conjunctiva and create a "pouch" into which the medication is instilled.

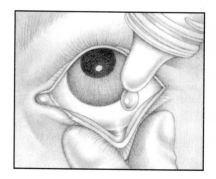

2 After drop instillation, gently close the eyelids and quickly apply light pressure at the inner corner of the eye near the bridge of the nose to prevent nasolacrimal outflow.

3 Encourage the patient to avoid factors, such as crying, that may increase lacrimal secretions.

How to instill eye ointment
Before applying an eye ointment, make sure you have the correct medication and that it's not outdated. Check the tube for the words "For ophthalmic use" or "For use in the eyes" because ophthalmic drugs are made with a special, nonirritating base suitable for the eye's sensitive tissues. Make sure the tube is at room temperature. Now you're ready to begin the procedure.

1 Darken the room if the light seems to irritate the patient. Then, position your patient on his back. Wash your hands and, if necessary, put on gloves. Take the time to reassure him and tell him what you're going to do. Explain that the ointment will temporarily cause blurred vision but that such blurring is normal and will disappear quickly.

2 Moisten a sterile gauze pad with normal saline solution. Working from the inner to the outer canthus, gently clean the patient's eyelids and lashes of any exudate, secretion, or old ointment. When you've finished, tilt his head back and urge him to relax. Remove the cap from the ointment tube, taking care not to contaminate either. Place the cap right side up on the table.

3 Ask the patient to look up and focus on a specific object. With one hand, place your index finger on the patient's cheekbone. Gently pull down on the skin to expose the conjunctival sac. Now, squeeze a thin ribbon of ointment along the conjunctival sac, starting at the inner canthus, as shown here. As you approach the outer canthus, rotate the tube to detach the ointment.

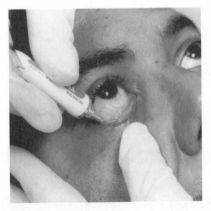

4 Release the patient's lower lid. Ask him to close his eyes for 1 to 2 minutes, so the medication can spread and be absorbed. Use a rayon ball or a tissue to gently wipe away any excess medication. Before replacing the cap on the tube, squeeze out a small drop of the medication and discard it. This may protect the remaining ointment from contamination.

5 Document the procedure, including your observations, in your nurse's notes.

MORGAN THERAPEUTIC LENS: TREATMENT GUIDELINES

INDICATION	INITIAL TREATMENT	CONTINUED TREATMENT
Ocular burn	Use Ringer's lactate solution with antibiotic and steroid added (as ordered). Give 500 ml, rapid free flow, by I.V. infusion set.	Continue flow at 50 ml/hour or 15 drops/minute until symptoms subside (24 to 72 hours).
Ocular injury from gasoline, detergent, or solvent	Give 500 ml Ringer's lactate solution, rapid free flow, by I.V. infusion set.	Continue infusion at slower rate, as indicated.
Foreign body sensation (but no visible foreign body)	Warm 20 ml sterile water for injection to body temperature and give by syringe (slow, gentle injection).	Repeat once, if indicated.
Severe ocular infection	Use Ringer's lactate solution with antibiotic and steroid added as ordered. Give 50 ml/hour or 15 drops/minute by I.V. infusion set.	Continue treatment for 70 hours; then repeat at 10-hour intervals, as indicated.
Preoperative antisepsis	Give 10 ml ocular antiseptic by syringe (slow, gentle injection).	Administer once.
Eyelid surgery	Give Ringer's lactate solution at 4 drops/minute.	Continue throughout procedure.

How to use the Morgan Therapeutic Lens

A patient who has a serious eye injury or infection may need immediate ocular lavage and medication to prevent complications or permanent eye damage. Inserted promptly after injury, the Morgan Therapeutic Lens minimizes damage and promotes healing. For many patients, it also relieves pain immediately. By providing continuous irrigation, it eliminates the need for repeated drop instillation.

The Morgan lens shown here consists of a molded scleral lens that connects to a 6" (15 cm) long silicone tube. One end of the tube attaches to a small, central hole in the lens; the other end, to a molded luer-lock adapter that you'll connect to a syringe or I.V. delivery system.

Fluid and medication, which flow through the tube at a controlled rate, can be stopped or changed without lens removal. The lens stays securely in place and flow remains constant even if the patient moves.

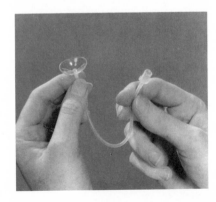

Before ocular surgery, the doctor may use the Morgan lens to flush the patient's conjunctiva. During eyelid surgery, he may use it to protect and irrigate the eye.

1 To avoid contact with drainage, put on gloves. Then instill a topical anesthetic.

2 To provide continuous lavage, attach the tube's adapter to the product-specific delivery set or an I.V. set containing the ordered solution. Then, begin the flow at the ordered rate.

NOTE Tubing shown here allows bilateral ocular lavage. To treat injury to both eyes, another lens would be attached to the other adapter.

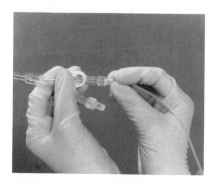

3 Ask the patient to look down, as shown. Insert the edge of the lens under the upper lid. Then tell her to look up as you retract her lower lid.

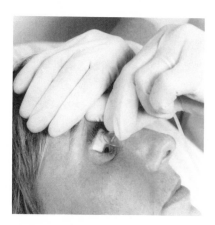

4 Release the lower lid over the lens. Securely in place, the lens now irrigates the eye continuously.

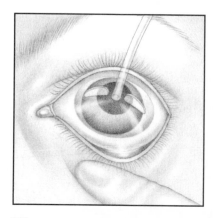

5 To prevent accidental lens displacement, tape the tube to the patient's forehead. Wipe off any excess solution with a towel.

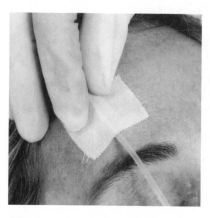

6 To remove the lens, ask the patient to look up as you retract the lower lid from the lens' lower border. Then, while holding this position, have the patient look down. Retract her upper lid and slide the lens out.

How to apply an eye patch

1 Wash your hands and put on gloves if necessary. Ask the patient to close both eyes. Use sterile gauze pads to fill his orbital space. This will provide a base for the patch and prevent the eyelid from opening.

2 Grasp the eye patch in the center, and place it over the gauze pads. Apply benzoin to his cheekbone.

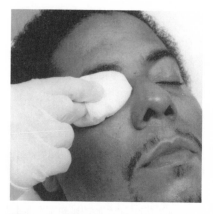

3 Secure the patch with two parallel strips of hypoallergenic tape. Work from the patient's midforehead to his cheekbone.

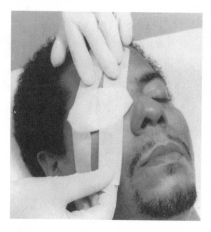

4 If the patient's eye requires extra protection, apply a black eye patch on top of the regular eye patch.

When it's time to instill the next dose of medication, remove the patch by loosening the tape from the forehead down. If you notice any drainage on the gauze or the patch, document your findings on the patient's chart.

Replace the gauze pads and patch with clean ones (if soiled) each time you instill medication.

Otic Administration

How to irrigate the ear

1 Seat the patient upright. Put on gloves if you see drainage or policy requires it. Examine the ear with an otoscope, noting color, blockage, and the patient's response to manipulation of the ear. Drape towels or bed-saver pads over her shoulder and around her neck. Clean the outer ear and auditory canal if necessary. Instruct her to hold an emesis basin or similar collection container under her affected ear.

2 Pull the auricle *up and back* to straighten the canal. With an ear syringe, instill approximately 50 ml warmed solution into the patient's ear. Direct the stream toward the *top* of the ear canal as shown, not toward the tympanic membrane. Don't occlude the auditory canal; allow the solution to flow out freely. Don't exert too much pressure or you could injure the ear canal.

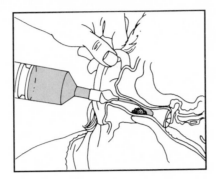

Check the solution as it drains into the basin. Look for wax and excess medication. Then, check the ear with an otoscope. If the ear canal still appears impacted, discard the drainage and repeat the procedure.

3 When you've removed all the softened wax and excess medication from the patient's ear, wash the skin around the ear with soap and water. Then, instruct her to lie on her affected side for several minutes to ensure complete drainage. Clean and dry the outer ear canal to prevent skin excoriation.

4 Document the procedure including the patient's response and the appearance of the drainage.

NURSING TIP Because this procedure may induce nausea or dizziness, it's helpful to schedule it either early or late in the day when the patient's stomach is empty.

How to administer ear drops

1 Before beginning the procedure, wash your hands. Check the medication label against the doctor's order. Warm the solution to body temperature by holding the bottle between your hands for 2 minutes. Never administer ear drops that aren't at body temperature, because this could cause vertigo.

Explain the procedure to your patient. Then, place her on her side so the affected ear is accessible. Examine the ear canal for drainage. If drainage is present, put on gloves and then gently clean the canal with a cotton-tipped applicator. Then check for new drainage and eardrum perforation. If you do not see drainage or perforation, proceed as follows.

2 Straighten the ear canal by gently pulling the auricle *up and back*. Remember, an infected ear is usually extremely painful. Be gentle.

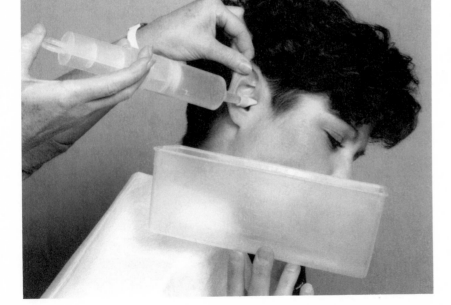

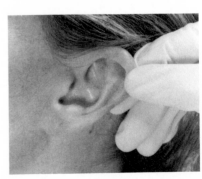

For a child under age 3, pull the auricle *down and back* as shown.

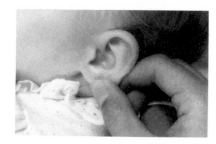

3 Taking care not to touch the ear with the dropper, instill the drops. Direct them along the side of the canal to avoid trapping any air in the ear. Then, hold the ear, as shown, until the medication disappears down the canal. Your patient will be able to tell you when the drops reach her tympanic membrane.

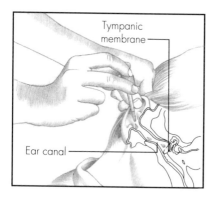

Tympanic membrane

Ear canal

4 Instruct your patient to remain on her side for about 5 minutes to keep the medication in the canal. Placing a medication-soaked cotton plug in her ear will also help (a dry cotton plug may absorb the medication). Then, clean and dry the outer ear and assist the patient to a comfortable position.

If both of the patient's ears require medication, let her stay on her side for 5 minutes, then repeat the procedure in her other ear.

Finally, document the procedure, as well as your observations, in your nurse's notes.

Nasal Administration

How to give nose drops to an adult

1 Confirm the medication order, and assemble the equipment: the bottle of medication, a medicine dropper, and tissues. Wash your hands and put on gloves if drainage is present or policy requires them. Explain the procedure to the patient and warn that he may taste the drops. If the patient has a sinus condition or can't sit up, place him in either the Proetz or the Parkinson position (see *Positioning the patient to treat the sinuses,* page 50). However, if the patient suffers from ordinary nasal congestion, seat him upright, with room to tilt his head back.

2 Draw enough medication into the dropper to instill the prescribed number of drops into the patient's nostrils. Avoid reinserting the dropper into the bottle, which increases the risk of contamination.

3 Open the patient's nostril completely by pushing up gently on the tip of his nose. Place the dropper about ⅓" (0.8 cm) inside the nostril. To avoid contaminating the dropper, don't let it touch the patient's nose.

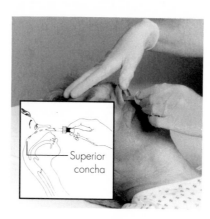

Superior concha

Direct the tip of the dropper toward the midline of the superior concha, as shown. This position will permit the medication to flow down the back of the patient's nose, not his throat.

Squeeze the dropper bulb to instill the correct number of drops into the nostril. Repeat the process in the other nostril, if ordered.

As you instill the drops, ask the patient to breathe through his mouth. This will suppress his urge to sniff, which could propel the medication into his sinuses.

4 Take care to prevent the patient from aspirating any medication. If he coughs, seat him upright and pat his back. Then, observe him closely for several minutes to see if any further respiratory problems develop.

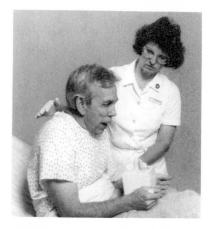

5 When you've instilled the correct number of drops, tell your patient to keep his head tilted back for about 5 minutes. Allow him to expectorate any medication that runs into his

POSITIONING THE PATIENT TO TREAT THE SINUSES

No matter which position you use, take care not to contaminate the dropper by touching the nostrils.

To instill medication in both the ethmoidal and the sphenoidal sinuses, place your patient in the Proetz position. Put him on his back, with his shoulders elevated and his head tilted back.

Use the Parkinson position to treat the maxillary and the frontal sinuses, located on each side of his face. This position is like the Proetz position, except the patient's head is tilted to one side instead of straight back.

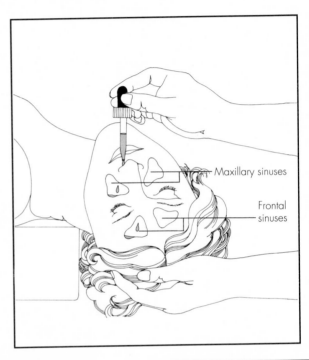

Sphenoidal sinus — Ethmoidal sinuses

Maxillary sinuses

Frontal sinuses

throat (it may have an unpleasant taste) and provide tissues. Clean the dropper with warm water and allow it to air-dry. Finally, document the entire procedure in your nurse's notes.

How to give nose drops to an infant

1 Check the medication order against the Kardex. Then, wash your hands and put on gloves if you notice drainage. Gather the following equipment: the bottle of medication, a medication dropper, and tissues.

Warm the medication by running warm water over the bottle for several minutes. Or warm it by carrying the bottle in your pocket for 30 minutes before administration.

Now, carefully position the infant so her head is tilted back on your arm, as shown.

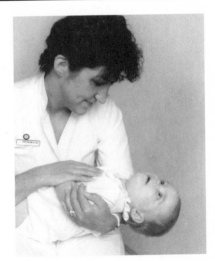

2 If the child is too large to hold in your arms, place him on his back, with a small pillow under his shoulders. Gently tilt his head back, supporting it between your forearm and your body, as shown. Restrain his arms and hands with one hand.

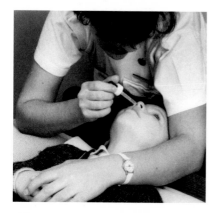

3 Draw the medication into the dropper. If possible, open the infant's nostrils by gently pushing up the tip of her nose. Instill the prescribed number of drops in the nostril. Avoid touching the nostril with the dropper.

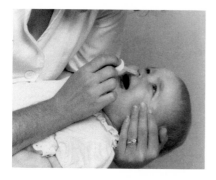

Repeat the process in the other nostril, if ordered.

After instilling the drops, keep the infant's head tilted back for 3 to 5 minutes (if possible). Stay alert for any sign of aspiration. If she begins to cough, sit her upright and pat her back until she's cleared her lungs.

If the patient has aspirated a large amount of medication, clear her respiratory tract with nasotracheal suctioning.

Finally, document the entire procedure and the infant's response.

NURSING TIP If you are administering decongestant (saline) drops, give them 20 minutes before mealtime to make eating easier. If you're giving them to an infant, gently suction the nostrils with an infant bulb syringe before administration to remove excess mucus, and suction again approximately 20 minutes after administration.

How to use an atomizer

1 Instruct the patient to read the medication label carefully so she knows the exact amount of medication to administer. Make sure she has tissues at hand. Then have the patient sit upright with her head tilted back.

If that position is uncomfortable, place the patient in the Proetz position.

2 Have the patient occlude one nostril with her finger as shown. Ask her to place the tip of the atomizer about ½"(1.3 cm) inside her open nostril. Direct her to point it straight up her nose, toward the inner corner of her eye. Caution her not to angle the atomizer downward, or the medication will run down her throat.

While she holds her breath, have her squeeze the atomizer once, quickly and firmly, using just enough force to coat the inside of her nose with medication. Too much force may send the medicine into her sinuses and cause a headache. Then, instruct her to spray again, if the instructions on the label order it. Repeat the procedure in the other nostril.

3 Instruct the patient to keep her head tilted back for several minutes, so the medication has time to work, and to avoid blowing her nose while waiting. To prevent overdosage, tell the patient not to use the atomizer more often than ordered.

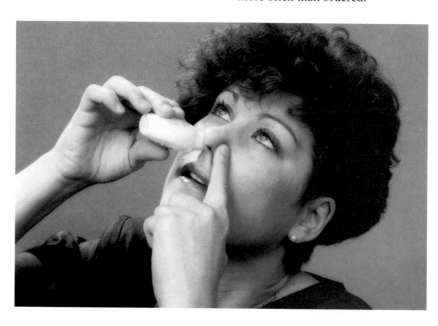

4 Have the patient rinse the atomizer tip with warm water to avoid contaminating the medication with nasal secretions.

5 Document the procedure and the patient's response.

How to use a nasal aerosol device (Turbinaire)

The Turbinaire is an aerosol device for intranasal application of metered doses of medication. It is used most frequently to treat inflamed nasal passages.

1 Instruct the patient to read the medication label so she knows the exact amount of medication to administer. Then, tell her to assemble the spray device by placing the stem of the medication cartridge in the plastic nasal adapter. (To insert a refill cartridge, she must first remove the protective cap from the stem.)

2 Ask the patient to gently blow her nose to remove excess mucus and clear the nostrils.

3 Tell her to shake the device well and remove the protective cap from the adapter tip.

4 Have the patient place the tip inside her nostril. Then, ask her to hold her breath, firmly press down once on the cartridge, and then release it. Encourage her to continue to hold her breath for several seconds afterward to avoid inhaling the mist.

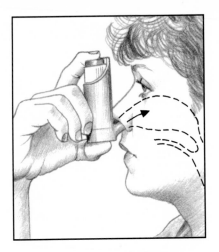

Now she may remove the adapter tip from her nostril and exhale through her mouth. If ordered, the patient should reinsert the adapter in the same nostril and spray again. Then tell her to shake the inhaler and repeat this procedure in the other nostril, if ordered.

> **Instruct the patient not to blow her nose for at least 2 minutes after each spray.**

5 Direct the patient to replace the protective cap on the adapter tip. Then, have her put the entire device in a plastic bag to keep it clean. Tell her to remove the medication cartridge once a day and thoroughly rinse the plastic adapter with warm water.

Document the procedure and observe the patient for signs of overdose or any other adverse reactions.

Laryngeal Administration

How to spray the mouth or throat

Gather this equipment: the ordered medication, a spoon, and tissues. Make sure the medication's warmed to 100° F (37.8° C) by setting its container in warm water. However, take care not to wet the spray nozzle.

1 Seat your patient upright and explain the procedure to him.

> If the patient can't sit up, ask the doctor if he can substitute another form of medication. Spraying the throat of a supine patient increases the risk of aspiration.

Put on gloves. Ask the patient to open his mouth. If you're administering an anesthetic (such as Chloraseptic), have the patient invert the bowl of a teaspoon over his tongue *before* you spray. This will keep his tongue from being numbed and help you see the irritated area of his throat. Instruct the patient to avoid inhaling as the medication is administered.

2 If you are using a spray pump, hold the nozzle just *outside* the patient's mouth and direct the medication toward his throat.

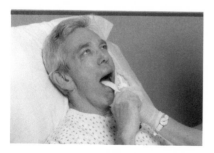

> If you've administered an anesthetic spray, warn the patient not to eat or drink for at least 1 hour. The anesthetic will inhibit his gag reflex and increase the risk of aspiration.

3 Document the procedure.

How to administer a mouthwash or gargle

1 Gather the solution, a drinking cup, an emesis basin, and tissues. Warm the solution by immersing its container in hot water. The container should be warm to the touch.

2 If the solution is used as a mouthwash, seat the patient upright or ask him to stand, if he's able. Instruct him to swish 1 to 4 oz (30 to 118 ml) of the solution around in his mouth, especially over his teeth and gums. Warn him not to swallow it. Instead, instruct him to spit it into the emesis basin. Hand him a tissue so he can wipe his mouth.

3 If the solution is used as a gargle, seat him upright with his head erect or tilted back slightly, as shown. Ask the patient to take a deep breath, then give him 1 oz of the solution and tell him to hold it in his mouth. Instruct him to exhale slowly to create the gargling action, but warn him not to inhale the solution. Tell him to spit the solution into the emesis basin and give him a tissue to wipe his mouth.

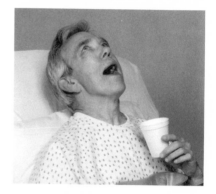

NURSING TIP If the doctor has ordered a medication like lidocaine hydrochloride (Xylocaine Viscous Solution), he may want you to instruct the patient to *swallow* the solution so it coats and soothes irritated throat tissue. If so, tell the patient not to eat or drink for a half hour afterward because the anesthetic will inhibit his gag reflex.

4 Document the procedure in your nurse's notes.

ADMINISTERING LOZENGES

If you're administering a lozenge (troche), instruct the patient to let it dissolve slowly in his mouth. Warn him not to fall asleep with the lozenge in his mouth, and remind him not to drink during or immediately after administration.

Note: Some lozenges contain sugar. If the patient's on a sugar-restricted diet, consult the doctor for a substitute medication.

Endotracheal Administration

Intermittent positive pressure breathing therapy

To help the patient who needs prolonged nebulization therapy several times a day either at home or in an acute care setting, the doctor may order intermittent positive pressure breathing (IPPB) therapy.

Check and record the patient's blood pressure, heart rate, and breath sounds to establish a baseline for comparison during and after therapy. Set the respirator at the prescribed pressure. Connect the mouthpiece to the respirator and ask the patient to inhale through it. Place the prescribed medication in the nebulizer cup. The respirator will automatically force medication into the patient's lungs until the preset pressure is reached. When the machine shuts off, tell the patient to remove the mouthpiece and exhale completely. Repeat the process for 10 or 15 minutes each session, as ordered.

After treatment, the patient may have episodes of coughing. Assure him that such coughing is both normal and beneficial.

PREPARING A PATIENT FOR IPPB THERAPY

• First, tell the patient that the equipment makes clicking, sighing noises; these can upset the patient who is not prepared for them.
• Explain the procedure to ensure the patient's cooperation.
• Have him sit in a chair with his feet on the floor. If he's on bedrest, place him in a high Fowler's position or sit him on the edge of the bed with his feet supported.
• Instruct him to practice breathing slowly and deeply through his mouth. Then, ask him to seal his lips tightly around the mouthpiece. Tell him to inhale slowly, allowing the equipment to do the work. When he exhales, have him breathe out around the mouthpiece. Assure him that the treatments will become easier with practice.
• Repeat the procedure until the nebulizer cup is empty (usually 15 to 20 minutes).
Nursing tip: Teach the patient to tap the side of the nebulizer cup periodically so that droplets can fall to the bottom.

NURSING CONSIDERATIONS: IPPB THERAPY

Stay alert for these danger signs and symptoms:
• sudden drop in blood pressure accompanied by increased heart rate (decreased venous return to the heart)
• nausea
• tremors or dizziness
• rapid, shallow respirations (respiratory alkalosis)
• distended abdomen (gastric insufflation)
• thickening of secretions (inadequate humidification)
• decreased respiratory rate (loss of hypoxic drive).

PORTABIRD II

The Portabird II is specifically designed for patients who must receive IPPB therapy at home.

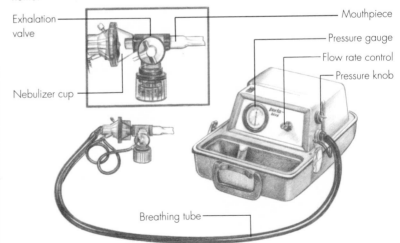

Exhalation valve — Mouthpiece — Pressure gauge — Flow rate control — Pressure knob — Nebulizer cup — Breathing tube

Endotracheal tube administration

In an emergency, if I.V. access isn't available, certain drugs can be administered through an endotracheal (ET) tube. This route allows uninterrupted resuscitation efforts and avoids such complications as coronary artery laceration, cardiac tamponade, or pneumothorax, which can occur with intracardial administration of emergency medication.

However, remember that after ET administration, a drug's duration of action is usually longer than after I.V. administration. That's because absorption is sustained in the alveoli, a phenomenon known as the depot effect. Therefore, expect to adjust repeat doses and continuous infusions to prevent adverse reactions.

How to give drugs through an endotracheal tube

1 Put on gloves. With your stethoscope, check placement of the ET tube as shown. Make sure the patient is supine and her head is level with or slightly higher than her trunk. Prepare the same initial dose that you would for an I.V. line, but dilute it in 5 to 10 ml of sterile water or normal saline solution. Diluting the drug increases the volume and allows a larger proportion of drug to leave the tube and contact lung tissue. If a prefilled syringe isn't available, use a standard 5- or 10-ml syringe.

Attach a positive-pressure oxygen delivery device (such as a hand-held resuscitation bag), quickly compress it three to five times, then remove the device.

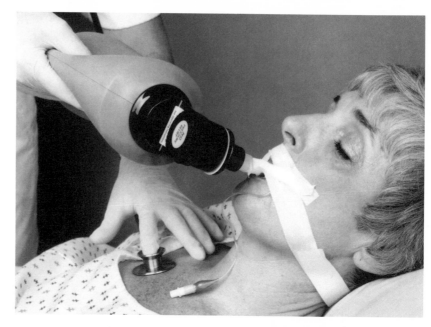

2 Remember to remove the needle before injecting medication into the ET tube. Inject the drug deep into the tube.

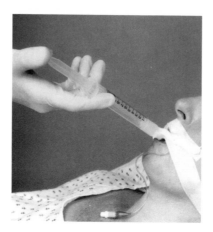

3 To prevent medication reflux, briefly place your thumb over the tube opening. Then reattach the resuscitation bag and quickly compress it five times to distribute the medication and oxygenate the patient.

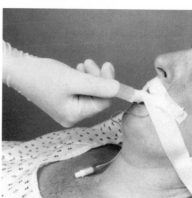

4 Document the procedure and monitor the patient's response. Be prepared: the onset of action may be quicker than it would be following I.V. administration. If the patient doesn't respond quickly, the doctor may order a repeat dose.

Endotracheal medication device

The endotracheal medication device offers an alternative to a syringe for delivering endotracheal medication.

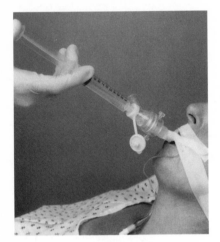

Usually used for bronchoscopy suctioning, this swivel adapter can be placed on the end of the endotracheal tube (A) and, while ventilation continues through a bag-valve device (B), endotracheal medication can be delivered with a needle through the closed stopcock (C).

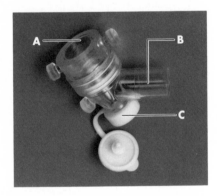

How to use a metered-dose inhaler

For a patient with respiratory disease, a metered-dose inhaler (MDI) provides a more effective alternative to hand-held nebulizers. The self-contained MDI unit consists of an

---

DRUGS DELIVERED BY MDI

Bronchodilators
- albuterol (Proventil, Ventolin)
- bitolterol (Tornalate)
- epinephrine (Medihaler-Epi, Primatene Mist)
- ipratropium (Atrovent)
- isoetharine (Bronkometer)
- isoproterenol (Isuprel, Medihaler-Iso)
- metaproterenol (Alupent, Metaprel)
- terbutaline (Brethaire)

Corticosteroids
- beclomethasone (Beclovent, Vanceril)
- flunisolide (AeroBid Inhaler)
- triamcinolone (Azmacort Inhaler)

---

inhaler attached to a unit-dose pressurized canister or capsule containing bronchodilators or steroids. The doctor may prescribe an MDI to treat chronic respiratory disease or acute conditions such as asthma attacks.

To use an MDI effectively, the patient must synchronize medication delivery with inhalations. If she can't (for example, because she has arthritis) she may need an extender (or spacer) to delay medication delivery (see How to Use an InspirEase Extender).

After you teach your patient to use an MDI, she can use it independently at home.

1 Instruct the patient to shake the MDI well to mix the medication and aerosol propellant. Then have her exhale fully and place the MDI mouthpiece between her lips as shown. Tell her to make sure neither her tongue nor her teeth block the opening.

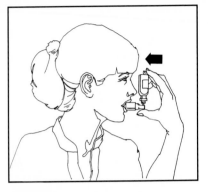

NOTE Some doctors recommend the open-mouth technique: the patient opens her mouth wide and positions the mouthpiece 2" to 4" (5.1 to 10.2 cm) from her lips.

2 Instruct the patient to press down on the canister while beginning a slow, deep inhalation as shown here. Inhaling slowly and deeply ensures maximum medication delivery. (The patient may need practice to master this step.)

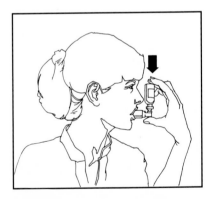

NOTE If the patient's using the open-mouth technique, have her release medication at the beginning of a 5-second inhalation.

3 After she has inhaled fully, tell her to hold her breath for 10 seconds, then to slowly exhale through her nose or pursed lips.

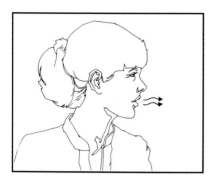

If the doctor has ordered two doses, the patient should wait 2 minutes before repeating the procedure.

How to use an InspirEase extender

Using valves or a reservoir bag, an extender delays medication delivery for patients who can't master MDI technique. The extenders currently available fit most MDIs. These photos show how to use the InspirEase extender and its components.

1 Tell the patient to connect the mouthpiece to the reservoir bag by aligning the inhaler's locking tabs with the bag's opening, as shown.

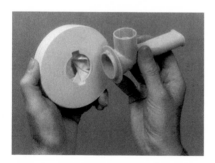

2 Have her gently untwist the reservoir bag to open it fully.

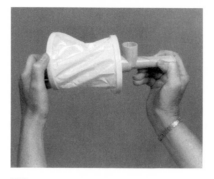

3 After shaking the MDI, place it snugly in the mouthpiece holder. Tell the patient to place the extender mouthpiece in her mouth and close her lips tightly around it. To release medication into the bag, have her press down on the MDI canister once or twice, as prescribed.

Next, tell her to inhale slowly through the mouthpiece.

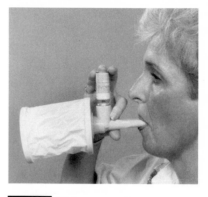

NOTE If the patient hears a whistling sound, she's inhaling too quickly.

4 Instruct the patient to continue inhaling until the bag collapses. Then have her hold her breath for 5 seconds and breathe out slowly into the bag. If appropriate, tell her to repeat the entire procedure.

BRETHANCER EXTENDER

The Brethancer is another extender that facilitates the use of conventional aerosol inhalers. It consists of three interlocking plastic components that telescope together for convenient carrying between uses. Easily opened with a single motion, the device traps medication in its middle portion for the patient to inhale. Tell the patient to breathe in as he depresses the canister.

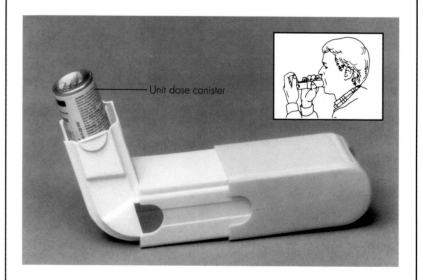

Unit dose canister

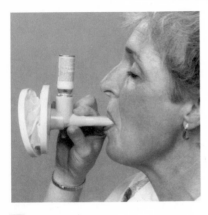

5 Instruct the patient to wash the mouthpiece in warm water and dry it completely. Tell her not to wash the reservoir bag.

How to use a turbo-inhaler

A type of MDI, the turbo-inhaler propels powder into the lung for systemic absorption. To teach a patient to use this drug delivery system, follow the guidelines below. Remind the patient to wash and dry his hands before unwrapping the capsule.

1 Have the patient hold the device so the white mouthpiece is on the bottom. Tell him to slide the gray sleeve all the way to the top.

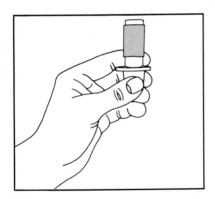

2 Ask him to open the mouthpiece by unscrewing its tip counterclockwise. He will see a small propeller on a stem inside.

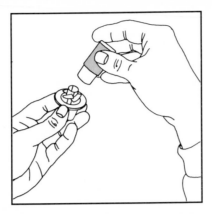

3 Observe the patient as he firmly presses the colored end of his medication capsule into the center of the propeller, as shown. Advise him to avoid overhandling the capsule, or it may soften.

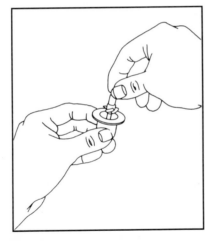

4 Instruct the patient to screw the device back together securely, holding it with the mouthpiece at the bottom, as shown. To puncture the capsule and release the medication, he must slide the gray sleeve all the way down, and then slide it up again. This step is done once.

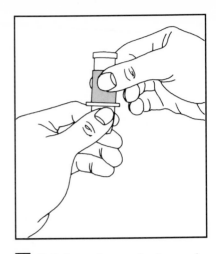

5 Tell the patient to check to make sure everything's secure, then hold the device away from his mouth, and exhale as much air as he can.

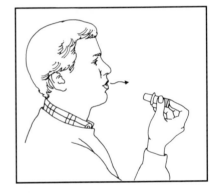

6 Ask him to tilt his head backward, place the mouthpiece in his mouth, and close his lips around it, as shown. Then, the patient should quickly inhale once to fill his lungs.

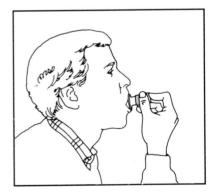

7 Encourage him to hold his breath for several seconds. Then, remove the device from his mouth, and have the patient exhale as much air as he can. Tell him to repeat steps 6 and 7 several times, until all the medication in the device is gone. Caution him to never exhale through the mouthpiece.

Remember to tell the patient to follow the doctor's instructions exactly, to never use more than four capsules a day, and to notify the doctor immediately if he experiences throat or chest irritation, coughing or choking, nasal congestion, dizziness, headache, or nausea.

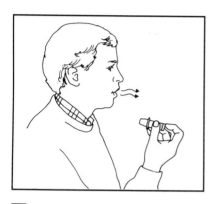

8 Tell the patient to discard the empty medication capsule, place the entire device in its metal can, and screw on the lid. At least once a week, he should remove the device from the can, take it apart, and rinse it thoroughly with warm water. Tell him to make sure it's completely dry before reassembling it, and to keep the capsules from deteriorating too rapidly by leaving them wrapped until needed.

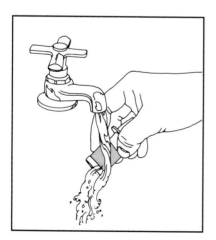

Parenteral Injection Equipment

Guide to syringes

Available from many manufacturers and in various sizes, syringes are made of reusable glass or disposable plastic. The latter type is the most widely used.

Syringes have a calibrated barrel with a plunger that fits inside. Depressing or pulling back on the plunger alters the space within the barrel, forcing its contents outward.

syringes (cartridges) include the needle and require a device to complete the unit for administration.

> **When handling the syringe, make sure you don't contaminate the plunger, the inside of the barrel, or the syringe tip. Maintaining sterility is an important aspect of giving injections correctly.**

Like oral medications, some parenteral medications are available in easy-to-use unit dose systems. Such prefilled syringes contain premeasured, ready-to-dispense doses enclosed in plastic cartridges that need only the attachment of a needle to be ready for use. Some prefilled

Outside barrel

Inside plunger

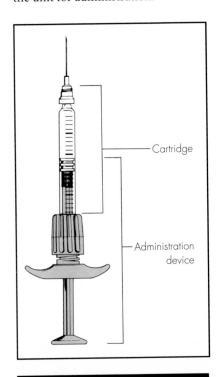

Cartridge

Administration device

> **When using a commercial prefilled syringe, administer precisely the dose prescribed. For example, if a 50 mg/ml cartridge is supplied but the patient's prescribed dose is 25 mg, you must administer only 0.5 ml (half of the volume contained in the cartridge). Be alert for potential medication errors whenever using premeasured dosage forms.**

SAFETY ADAPTATION: NEEDLE SHIELD

Because of the potential for transmission of bloodborne diseases from patients to staff, manufacturers have adapted needles and syringes to help prevent needle-stick injuries. For example, a new hypodermic safety device built into the syringe-needle combination eliminates the need for recapping the needle.

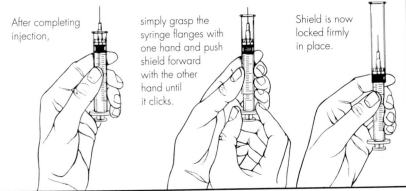

After completing injection,

simply grasp the syringe flanges with one hand and push shield forward with the other hand until it clicks.

Shield is now locked firmly in place.

SELECTING NEEDLES

Needles are available in various lengths, diameters (gauges), and bevel designs. The illustrations below will help you select the correct needle for the injection route you're using.

Intradermal

For an intradermal injection, select a needle $3/8$" to $5/8$" (1 to 1.5 cm) in length, 25G to 26G in diameter, with a short bevel.

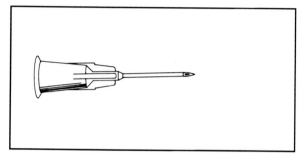

Subcutaneous

For a subcutaneous injection, select a needle $5/8$" to $7/8$" (1.5 to 2 cm) in length, 24G to 27G in diameter, with a medium bevel.

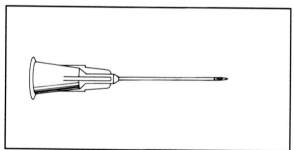

Intramuscular

For an intramuscular injection, select a needle 1" to 3" (2.5 to 7.5 cm) in length, 19G to 23G in diameter, with a medium bevel.

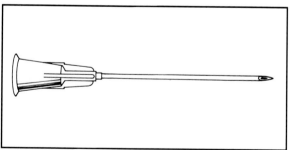

Intravenous

For an intravenous injection, select a needle 1" to 3" in length, 16G to 21G in diameter, with a long bevel.

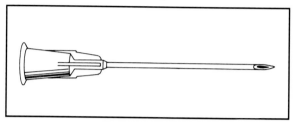

Butterfly

Steel winged needle used for intravenous infusion, 16G to 21G in diameter, with a short bevel.

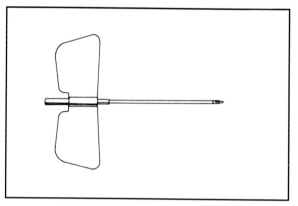

Noncoring (Huber) needle

For use with venous access ports, it has a deflected tip that won't damage the port.

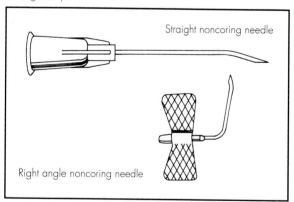

Straight noncoring needle

Right angle noncoring needle

SAFETY ADAPTATION: I.V. ACCESS SYSTEM

Another safety modification is the needleless I.V. access system, in which a blunt-ended cannula is attached to the syringe, requiring a product-specific rubber injection site. This site has a preestablished slit that can open and reseal immediately.

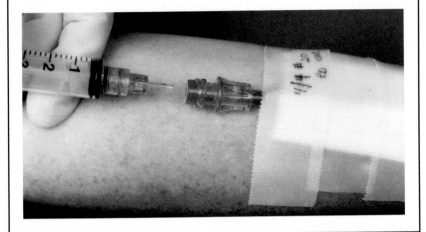

How to prepare medication for injection

The ordered medication may be a liquid or a powder. Liquid medications come in glass ampules or vials and are ready to draw into a syringe. If administering a toxic drug such as cyclophosphamide (Cytoxan), wear gloves.

If the medication comes in a vial, clean the stopper with alcohol. Pull back the plunger until the amount of air in the barrel equals the amount of medication ordered. Then, insert the needle into the vial stopper, inject the air, and withdraw the medication.

If the medication comes in a glass ampule, score the neck of the ampule with a razor blade if it's not pre-scored. Then, wrap the ampule in a semidry alcohol pad. Grasp the ampule and snap off the top. Place a filter needle in the open ampule and withdraw the prescribed dose.

If the medication comes in a powder, you will have to reconstitute it. To do this, you will need the medication, a vial of compatible diluent, an 18G filter needle and syringe, and an alcohol pad.

After you have assembled the equipment, remove the protective cap from the diluent vial and wipe the stopper with alcohol. Then, follow the steps below:

1 Inject an amount of air equal to the recommended amount of diluent into the diluent vial, as shown.

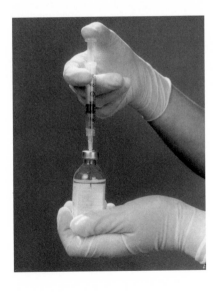

2 Draw the recommended amount of diluent into the needle and syringe.

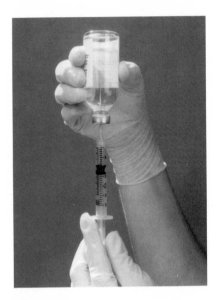

3 Wipe the medication bottle's stopper with alcohol, and inject the diluent into the bottle.

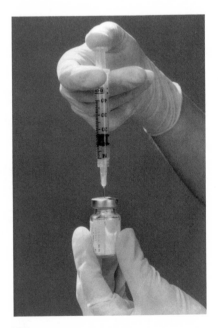

4 Mix the medication and diluent, then draw up the reconstituted medication.

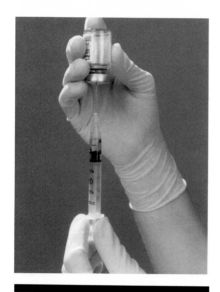

Intradermal Administration

Learning about intradermal administration

Intradermal injection (injection into the outer layer of the skin) is usually performed to:
• determine sensitivity to a specific antigen and to stimulate an immune response
• identify antibodies that have developed against pathogens, such as the tubercle bacillus
• infiltrate the skin with an anesthetic before venipuncture.

NOTE Don't expect an immediate reaction. The capillaries of the dermis have a slower absorption rate than subcutaneous tissue or muscle.

In patients who are hypersensitive to the test antigen, intradermal injection can cause a severe anaphylactic response. This requires immediate injection of epinephrine and other emergency resuscitation procedures. Be especially alert for anaphylactic response after giving a test dose of penicillin or tetanus antitoxin.

PREPARING FOR INJECTION

Injecting a medication incorrectly may damage nerves, tissue, or blood vessels, or introduce bacteria. To avoid such complications:
• Select the site carefully to avoid damaging nerves and vessels.
• Avoid areas that are inflamed or have lesions, hair, or birthmarks.
• Use only sterile needles and syringes and avoid contamination.
• Select the right length needle for the injection and the patient's size.
• Check for blood backflow to confirm placement in a vein before I.V. injection. For S.C., I.M., and intradermal injections, if you see blood in the syringe barrel, remove the needle. Then select another site and try again with a new needle.
• Have someone nearby to help restrain the patient, if necessary.
• Establish a site rotation plan for frequent injections; record it on the patient's Kardex.
• Discard needle and syringe according to universal precautions.

INTRADERMAL INJECTION SITES

Intradermal injection is commonly performed on the ventral forearm, but can also be given at the sites shown here if, for example, the skin of the arm is irritated or burned. These alternative sites are lightly pigmented, thinly keratized and usually hairless. These characteristics allow easier evaluation of injection reactions.

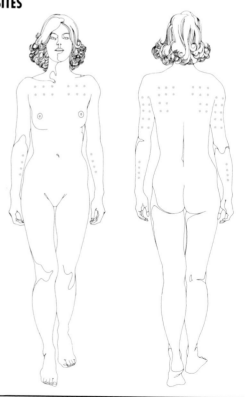

How to inject medication intradermally

1 Assemble your equipment: the medication, a 1 ml tuberculin syringe, a 26G ⅝" (1.5 cm) needle, acetone, a 4" × 4" gauze pad, several alcohol pads, and gloves. If your patient has a history of drug allergy, you'll also need normal saline solution or an allergy test diluent, plus another needle and syringe, to make a control wheal.

If necessary, attach the needles to the syringes. Check the medication to make sure it's not outdated or contaminated. If the medication is okay, draw it into one of the syringes. Then cap the syringe and bring all of the equipment to the bedside.

Tell the patient what you're about to do. Position the arm with the ventral forearm exposed and supported on a flat surface, and the elbow flexed. The patient may be sitting or lying down for this procedure, as long as he's comfortable.

2 Put on gloves. Locate the patient's antecubital space. Then measure several finger widths away from it in the direction of the hand, ending about a handbreadth away from the wrist. Avoid any hairy or blemished areas, which could make reading the test result difficult.

Defat the skin with acetone and a gauze pad, beginning at the center of the site and moving outward in a circular motion. Then, using a similar motion, prepare the skin with an alcohol pad. Never use a disinfectant like povidone-iodine (Betadine), which will discolor the skin, and avoid rubbing too vigorously, which can cause irritation. Either action could hinder reading of the test.

Allow the skin to dry thoroughly. If you inject while the skin is wet, you can introduce antiseptic into the dermis, which could affect test results.

3 Hold the patient's forearm and stretch the skin with your thumb, as shown. With your other hand, hold the syringe between your thumb and forefinger, and rest the plunger against the heel of your palm. Expel any air in the needle.

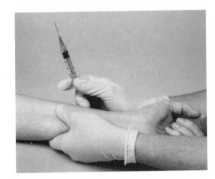

4 Position the syringe so that the needle is almost flat against the patient's skin. Make sure the bevel of the needle is up. Then, insert the needle by pressing it against the skin until you meet resistance. Advance the needle through the epidermis so that the point of the needle is visible through the skin. Stop when it's resting ⅛" (3 mm) below the skin's surface, between the epidermis and the dermis.

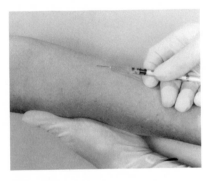

5 Slowly and gently inject the medication. Expect to feel some resistance, which confirms that the needle is correctly placed. If the plunger moves too freely, you've inserted the needle too deeply. Withdraw it slightly and try again. When you've finished injecting the medica-

tion, leave the needle in place momentarily. Watch for a small white blister or wheal to form, about ¼" (6 mm) in diameter.

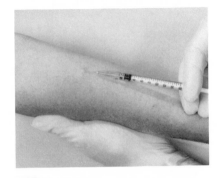

6 When the wheal appears, withdraw the needle and apply gentle pressure to the site. Don't massage it, because doing so may interfere with test results.

Now make a control wheal as shown. Draw up normal saline solution or allergy test diluent in the second syringe. Inject it into the patient's other arm or another site on the arm being tested, using the same procedure.

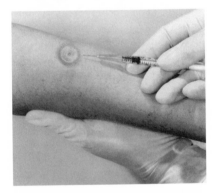

7 Document the name of the medication and the amount administered. If the patient has an allergic reaction within 30 minutes, notify the doctor. In most cases, a reaction occurs within 48 to 72 hours. For test result guidelines, see How to Read a Diagnostic Skin Test.

How to read a diagnostic skin test

1 The area around the injection site should feel hard to the touch (indurated) before you begin your reading. Record the extent of induration in millimeters. Also measure the extent of erythema, if present. But remember, erythema without hardening is insignificant.

When testing for tuberculosis, use the test result scale shown to evaluate the results. Because different tests use different scales, always check the package insert that comes with the medication.

2 Examine the site. If the induration is smaller than ¹/₄" (5 mm) in diameter, consider the results negative.

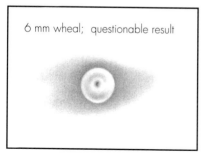
4 mm wheal; negative result

3 If the induration is ¹/₄" to ³/₈" (5 to 9 mm) in diameter, consider the results doubtful and perform another test

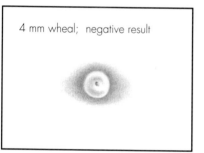
6 mm wheal; questionable result

4 If the induration is greater than ³/₈" (9 mm) or more, the result is positive.

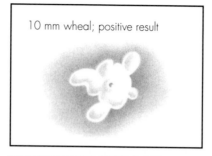
10 mm wheal; positive result

Subcutaneous Administration

Learning about subcutaneous administration

Give a medication subcutaneously when you want it to take effect slowly. Most subcutaneous medications are isotonic, nonirritating, nonviscous, and soluble. They are absorbed through both adipose and connective tissue.

Subcutaneous injection may be ordered if:
• the medication is more effective if absorbed through subcutaneous tissue
• the patient can't or won't swallow
• the patient can't take anything by mouth because of vomiting or the need for gastric suctioning
• the medication's action would be destroyed by gastrointestinal secretions
• the medication would irritate the gastrointestinal tract
• the patient's veins don't allow venous access
• continuous slow infusion is desired. (Hypodermoclysis is the infusion of fluid into subcutaneous tissue through an intravenous set.)

Subcutaneous injection should be avoided if:
• the patient is in shock
• the patient has occlusive vascular disease with poor perfusion
• the patient's skin tissue is grossly adipose, edematous, burned, hardened, or swollen at all the common injection sites
• the patient's skin is diseased
• the patient's skin was damaged by previous injections
• the drug is not appropriate for subcutaneous administration.

You can give a subcutaneous injection in any part of the body that has relatively few sensory nerve endings and no bones or large blood vessels near the surface.

When selecting an injection site, make sure it has a fat fold of at least 1" (2.5 cm) when you pinch the area between your thumb and forefinger. You'll find subcutaneous tissue abundant in well nourished, well hydrated patients and sparse in frail, cachexic, or dehydrated patients.

Absorption rate

Because blood is minimal in subcutaneous tissue, the absorption rate, which is chiefly influenced by blood flow, is usually slow. But a few medications defy this rule. Heparin and some other drugs are absorbed through the subcutaneous tissue as rapidly as through intramuscular tissue.

Several other factors also influence absorption from subcutaneous sites:
• Trauma of injection releases histamine into subcutaneous tissue, which decreases blood flow and slows absorption.
• Physical exertion increases blood flow in subcutaneous tissue, speeding up absorption.
• Normal connective tissue prevents medication from spreading indiscriminately and slows absorption. This process is altered by the enzyme hyaluronidase, which breaks down hyaluronic acid, a basic substance in

SUBCUTANEOUS ADMINISTRATION SITES

The most commonly used subcutaneous sites are the outer aspects of the arms and thighs. Less common sites include the lower abdomen, above the iliac crest, and the upper back.

connective tissue. As the hyaluronidase level in the medication increases, so do the rates of absorption and
diffusion.
• A highly soluble medication is
absorbed more rapidly than a less
soluble one.

Complications
Subcutaneous injections are relatively
safe, but can cause certain complications. For example, an injection of
concentrated or irritating solutions
can cause sterile abscesses to form as
a result of natural immune response.
Repeated injections into the same site
can cause lipodystrophy, atrophy of
the subcutaneous tissue. This is an
especially difficult problem in
patients with diabetes, who require
daily injections of insulin. For such
patients, rotating the injection sites
can help minimize tissue damage.

How to inject medication subcutaneously

1 Gather the following equipment:
the prescribed medication, several
alcohol pads, a 1 ml syringe with a ⅝"
(1.5 cm) needle attached, and an
assortment of other needles up to
27G in diameter and ½" to 1" (1.3 to
2.5 cm) in length.
   Next, select the injection site (the
deltoid is shown). To locate it, hold
the patient's arm firmly by his side,
inner aspect up. Then measure one
handbreadth down from the shoulder and a third of the way around to
the outer aspect of the arm. Explain
the procedure to the patient as you
work.

2 To determine the exact needle
size, use your thumb and forefinger
to form a fold of skin at the site.

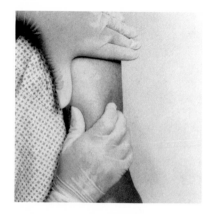

   Measure from the fold's base to its
crest. If the fold measures more or
less than ⅝" (1.5 cm), remove the ⅝"
needle from the syringe and replace it
with one that's closer to the correct
length. You'll probably need a ½"
(1.3 cm) needle for a child or a thin
patient, and a ⅞" or 1" (2 or 2.5 cm)
needle for an overweight patient.
   By using the correct size needle,
you minimize the risk of missing the
subcutaneous tissue and spare your
patient unnecessary pain.

3 Examine the medication. Make
sure it's not contaminated or outdated. Next, remove the metal cap on
the vial and expose the rubber stopper. Use an alcohol pad to clean the
rubber top. Then remove the cap
from the needle and pierce the rubber stopper in the center with the
needle tip. Inject a volume of air into
the vial that's equal to the volume of
medication you wish to extract. Now,
holding the syringe at eye level, withdraw the prescribed amount of drug.
If air bubbles accumulate as you
withdraw the drug, tap the barrel of
the syringe and reinject the air into
the vial. Continue this process until
the desired dose is extracted from the

vial. Remove the needle from the vial
and, if you are using a multi-dose
vial, store it according to product-
specific instructions.
   Pull back on the plunger to introduce a 0.2 to 0.3 cc air bubble into
the syringe barrel. Later, when you
inject the medication, this bubble will
help seal it in the subcutaneous tissue.

4 Clean the site with an alcohol
pad, beginning at the center of the
site and moving outward with a circular motion. Allow the skin to dry
completely before you proceed. If the
skin is still wet when you inject the
medication, you may introduce alcohol into the subcutaneous tissue.

5 Grasp the skin firmly, as shown.
This elevates the subcutaneous tissue
and prevents the needle from entering the wrong skin layer. Position the
needle bevel up. If injecting with a ½"
(1.3 cm) needle, hold it at a 90-
degree angle to the skin. If you're
using a ⅝" (1.5 cm) or longer needle,
hold it at a 45-degree angle. Insert
the needle with one quick motion.
Once the needle is inserted, release
your grasp on the patient's skin. If
you don't, you'll inject into the compressed tissue, which will irritate
nerve fibers and cause discomfort.

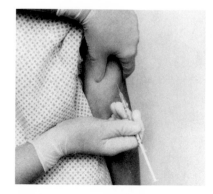

6 Pull back slightly on the plunger
to check needle placement. If you get

blood backflow, quickly withdraw the needle and place an alcohol pad over the site. If the blood discolors the contents of the syringe, discard everything and begin again. However, if blood backflow is minimal, simply replace the needle with a sterile one and insert it at a new site.

If there's no blood backflow, begin injecting the medication slowly. Never inject rapidly; doing so will put pressure on the tissue and cause pain.

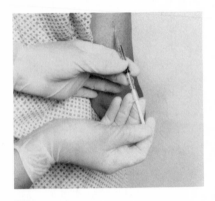

7 When you've finished injecting, place an alcohol pad over the site. Then withdraw the needle at the same angle used for insertion. As you do, use the pad to apply pressure to the site. Applying pressure will help seal the site and prevent seepage of the medication. Next, use a clean alcohol pad to massage the site. This will help distribute the medication and promote its absorption by dilating the blood vessels in the area and increasing blood flow.

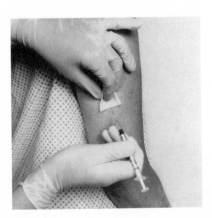

8 Document the procedure and the patient's response to it. Include the name of the prescribed drug, its dosage, route, site, time of administration, and your initials. Afterward, dispose of all equipment according to policy.

How to mix insulins in one syringe using multidose vials

Gather equipment for subcutaneous injection (see How to Inject Medication Subcutaneously, page 67). Wash your hands and remove the protective metal caps from the unopened vials. Use alcohol pads to clean the rubber stoppers of both vials.

1 Remove the cap from the needle and inject a volume of air equal to the volume of drug needed into the modified insulin vial to equalize the

pressure. Do not extract the drug or allow the needle tip to touch the medication. Remove the needle and syringe.

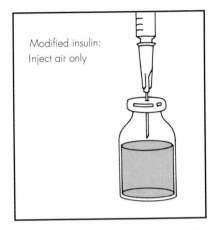

Modified insulin: Inject air only

2 Inject a volume of air equal to the desired volume of regular insulin into the regular insulin vial and, while holding the vial at eye level,

---

DIAL-A-DOSE SYSTEM

The Dial-a-Dose delivery system offers an alternative to the conventional syringe and vial system of insulin administration.

The device is designed to resemble a fountain pen and uses a 1.5 ml cartridge of insulin delivered by a push-button plunger mechanism.

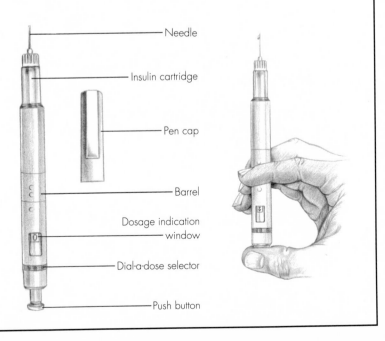

- Needle
- Insulin cartridge
- Pen cap
- Barrel
- Dosage indication window
- Dial-a-dose selector
- Push button

GUIDELINES FOR INSULIN ADMINISTRATION

• To establish more consistent blood levels, rotate insulin injection sites within anatomic regions. Absorption varies from one region to another. Preferred insulin injection sites are the arms, abdomen, thighs, and buttocks.

• Make sure the type of insulin, dose, and syringe are correct.

• Some insulins can be mixed together to fine-tune their onset, peak, and duration of action, helping the patient to achieve better glucose control.

• When combining insulins, be sure they are compatible.

• Prompt insulin zinc suspension (Semi-lente) *cannot* be mixed with isophane insulin suspension (NPH). Follow institution policy as to which insulin to draw up first.

• Insulin zinc suspension (Lente), prompt insulin zinc suspension (Semi-lente), and extended insulin zinc suspension (Ultralente) are compatible in any proportion.

• Most regular insulins can be mixed with other insulins. But do not mix human zinc suspension insulin (Velo-sulin Human) with insulin zinc suspension (Lente) because their buffering systems aren't compatible.

• Don't mix insulins of different purities or origins.

• Regular insulin is compatible with protamine zinc insulin suspension (PZI), but this mixture isn't usually recommended because its glycemic effects are unpredictable.

• Before drawing up insulin suspension, gently roll and invert the bottle to ensure even particle distribution. Cloudiness, discoloration or white "strings" usually indicate contamination. Discard the vial and use a new one. *Do not* shake the bottle, because this can cause foaming, changing the potency and altering the dose.

GUIDELINES FOR HEPARIN ADMINISTRATION

To inject heparin, follow the procedure for any subcutaneous injection, except for these considerations:

• The preferred site for heparin injections is the lower abdominal fat pad, 2" (5.1 cm) beneath the umbilicus between the iliac crests. Injecting heparin into this area, which is not involved in muscular activity, reduces the risk of local capillary bleeding. Always rotate the injection site from one side to the other.

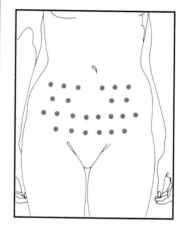

• Do not administer any injections within 2" of a scar, a bruise, or the umbilicus.

• Pinch a 1/2" (1.3 cm) fold of tissue between your thumb and forefinger, and insert the needle into the fold at a 90-degree angle. Using this technique will minimize heparin's irritating qualities. Don't apply ice unless policy permits it and you have a doctor's order.

Important: Do not aspirate to check for blood return because this may cause bleeding into tissue at the site.

• Do not rub or massage the site after injection. Rubbing can cause localized, minute hemorrhages or bruises.

---

extract the prescribed amount of regular insulin.

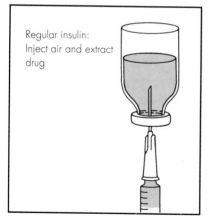

Regular insulin:
Inject air and extract drug

3 Insert the needle into the modified insulin vial and, holding the vial at eye level, extract the desired volume. (By withdrawing the regular insulin first, you avoid contaminating it with longer acting insulin containing globulin or protamine. The contaminated regular insulin would have an unpredictable onset of action.) Cap the needle and store the vials as recommended by the manufacturer.

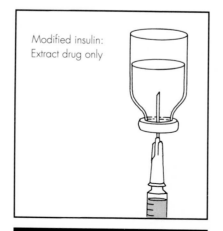

Modified insulin:
Extract drug only

Intramuscular Administration

INTRAMUSCULAR INJECTION SITES

Intramuscular injection is appropriate in the ventrogluteal, deltoid, dorsogluteal, vastus lateralis, and rectus femoris muscles. The absorption rate at each of these sites is about the same. Study the following illustrations to determine which site is best for a patient.

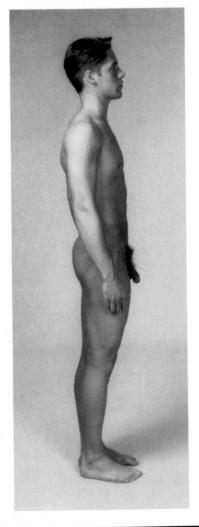

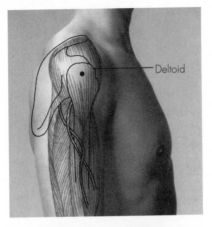

DELTOID

This site is seldom used because the muscle is small and can accommodate only small volumes of medication. It's also dangerously near the radial nerve.

For deltoid injection, the patient may sit upright or lie flat, with arms apart.

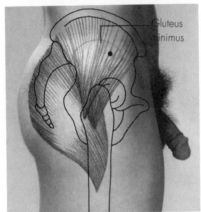
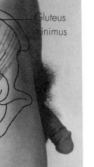

VENTROGLUTEAL

This site, which can be used for all patients, is desirable because it is relatively free from large nerves and fatty tissue and is remote from the rectum, which minimizes the risk of contamination.

For ventrogluteal injection, position the patient on his back or side.

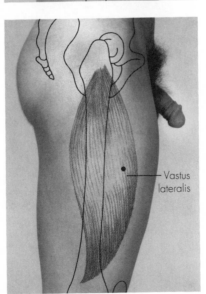

VASTUS LATERALIS

The vastus lateralis is used for all patients and is especially recommended for children. It's well developed and has few major blood vessels and nerves. Position the patient in bed sitting up or lying flat.

INTRAMUSCULAR INJECTION SITES *continued*

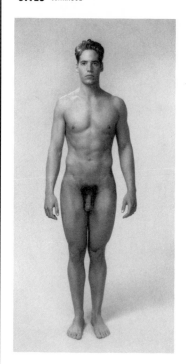

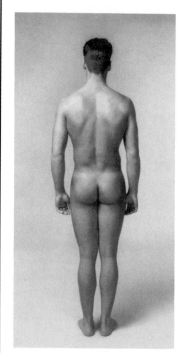

RECTUS FEMORIS

The rectus femoris is most often used for self-injection because of its accessibility. Position the patient in bed sitting up or lying flat.

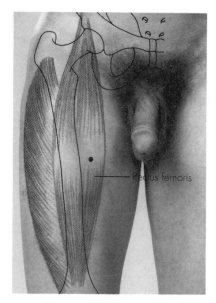

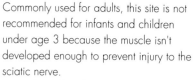

DORSOGLUTEAL

Commonly used for adults, this site is not recommended for infants and children under age 3 because the muscle isn't developed enough to prevent injury to the sciatic nerve.

For dorsogluteal injection, position the patient flat on the stomach, with toes pointed inward and arms apart and flexed toward the head.

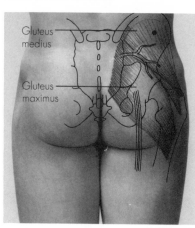

INTRAMUSCULAR INJECTIONS: PROS AND CONS

Intramuscular absorption is similar to but more rapid than subcutaneous absorption because of increased blood flow to the muscles. For example, aqueous medications are absorbed from a muscle site within 10 to 30 minutes; absorption takes more than 30 minutes from a subcutaneous site. Keep in mind, however, that not all intramuscular medications take effect at the same rate.

Give medication by the intramuscular route when you want to:
• administer aqueous suspensions, solutions in oil, or medications that are insoluble in oral form.
• administer parenteral medication in large doses (up to 5 ml).
• administer medication to a patient who's uncooperative, unconscious, or unable to swallow.
• avoid loss of drug effects from vomiting or gastric activity.
• achieve a rapid effect.
• ensure long-term absorption by forming a medication deposit.

The advantages of using the intramuscular route over other parenteral routes are that muscles contain more blood vessels and have fewer sensory nerve endings. However, the oral and I.V. routes are preferred for administration of drugs that are poorly absorbed by muscle tissue, such as phenytoin (Dilantin), digoxin (Lanoxin), chlordiazepoxide (Librium), diazepam (Valium), and haloperidol (Haldol). The potential risks of the intramuscular route include:
• damage to blood vessels, resulting in bleeding or improper routing of medication.
• damage to nerves, causing paralysis or unnecessary pain.
• damage to bone.

How to inject medication intramuscularly

1 Wash your hands. (Remember to maintain sterile technique throughout the procedure.) Then, gather your equipment: medication, diluent, syringe, appropriate size needle, several alcohol pads, and gloves.

Examine the medication vial. Make sure it's not outdated or contaminated. Then explain to the patient what you're going to do and provide privacy.

2 Prepare the medication. Then wipe the stopper on the medication vial with alcohol. Attach the needle to the syringe and insert it into the stopper. Draw up the correct amount of the drug, then draw up 0.2 to 0.3 cc of air. This air bubble will help clear the medication from the needle when you inject. It will also prevent seepage of the medication from the injection site afterward.

3 Assume you decide to use the vastus lateralis site for the injection. To expose the site, position the patient on her back. Gently tap at the site, as shown. This will stimulate the nerve endings and minimize pain when the needle is inserted.

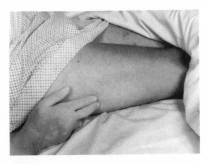

4 Clean a 2" (5 cm) area around the injection site, moving outward from the center in a circular motion. This will reduce the risk of introducing pathogens into the tissue when you penetrate the skin with the nee-

dle. Place the alcohol pad between two of your fingers for later use. Let the skin dry before you inject so you don't force any alcohol into the subcutaneous tissue, causing pain.

5 With one hand, stretch the skin taut around the injection site. This makes needle insertion easier and displaces subcutaneous tissue, which helps disperse the medication.

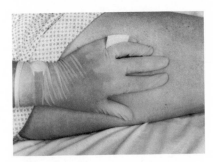

6 Use your other hand to hold the syringe. Keep it horizontal until you're ready to inject, as shown. Doing so will prevent gravity from altering the position of the plunger. Insert the needle at a 90-degree angle, with a quick, dartlike thrust (expect to feel some resistance). This quick thrust facilitates needle entry and minimizes pain.

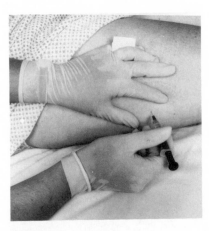

7 Gently pull back on the plunger to confirm needle placement. If blood appears in the syringe, you may have punctured a vein. With-

draw the needle, replace it with a new one, and try again. If no blood appears, continue to the next step.

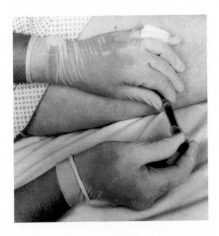

NURSING CONSIDERATIONS: I.M. INJECTIONS

Intramuscular injections can traumatize local muscle cells, causing elevated serum levels of such enzymes as creatine phosphokinase (CPK) that can be confused with the elevated enzyme levels resulting from damage to cardiac muscle, as in myocardial infarction (MI). To differentiate between skeletal and cardiac muscle damage, diagnostic tests for suspected MI must identify the CPK isoenzyme specific to cardiac muscle (CPK-MB-CPK_2) and must include tests for lactic dehydrogenase (LDH) and aspartate aminotransferase (AST).

If measuring these blood levels is critical, suggest that the doctor switch to I.V. administration (with dosage adjustments).

8 Inject the medication at a slow, even rate. If you force it, you'll cause unnecessary pain and improper drug distribution.

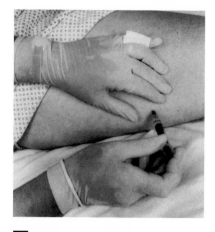

9 When you've finished injecting, withdraw the needle rapidly. Use an alcohol pad to apply pressure to the site. As you continue to apply pressure, massage the site with a circular motion. This will distribute the medication over a greater area.

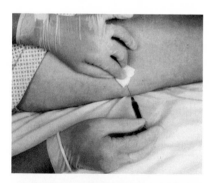

> **Don't massage the site when you want slow absorption or when you're injecting an extremely irritating medication, such as cefazolin (Ancef).**

Watch for adverse reactions immediately after the injection and up to 30 minutes afterward. Docu-

ment medication, route, site, time, patient's reaction, and your initials. Finally, discard the equipment according to policy and universal precautions. Be sure to wash your hands afterward.

How to give I.M. injections to infants and toddlers

Generally, the principles of intramuscular administration in children are the same as in adults. The recommended changes in procedure are related to differences in muscle mass. The younger the child, the less developed the muscle. For example, the gluteal muscles, which develop with walking, are never developed enough for safe intramuscular administration in children under age 3, or in children who have not been walking for at least a year. To prevent injury to the sciatic nerve by injection into the small gluteal muscle, the recommended intramuscular sites are the vastus lateralis (anterior thigh), and, if it is sufficiently developed, the deltoid.

For intramuscular injection in children, use a ½" to 1" (1.3 to 2.5 cm), 25G to 27G needle. The volume injected should not exceed 0.5 ml in an infant, or 1 ml in a small child (see *Maximum intramuscular solution volumes for children,* page 74). Another important difference is that all children under age 5 should be restrained during intramuscular injection. Even the most cooperative child may be unable to hold still during the injection and could sustain muscle damage.

For injection into the anterior thigh, position the child as shown. Don't ask a parent to help you restrain the child; because pain is associated with this procedure, the parent may be unable to resist moving. Instead, proceed as follows:

Put on gloves if necessary. Grasp the chosen leg firmly below the knee with your nondominant hand and lean across the child's torso with your upper body, being careful not to put too much pressure on the child's chest. Now with your dominant hand, administer the injection. Immediately afterward, hand the child to the parent for comforting and praise him for cooperation.

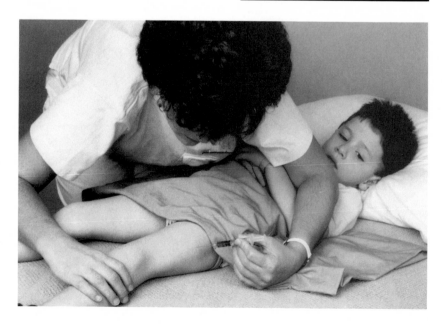

MAXIMUM INTRAMUSCULAR SOLUTION VOLUMES FOR CHILDREN

For a child, the amount of solution that you can administer safely via intramuscular injection depends on several factors—most important, the child's age and the injection site. The following chart lists the maximum recommended volumes of injections in the various muscle groups for children of different ages.

MUSCLE GROUP	AGE				
	Birth to 1¹/₂ years	**1¹/₂ to 3 years**	**3 to 6 years**	**6 to 15 years**	**15 years to adult**
Deltoid	Not recommended	0.5 ml (Not recommended unless other sites aren't available)	0.5 ml	0.5 ml	1 ml
Gluteus maximus	Not recommended	1 ml (Not recommended unless other sites aren't available)	1.5 ml	1.5 to 2 ml	2 to 2.5 ml
Ventrogluteal	Not recommended	1 ml (Not recommended unless other sites aren't available)	1.5 ml	1.5 to 2 ml	2 to 2.5 ml
Vastus lateralis	0.5 to 1 ml	1 ml	1.5 ml	1.5 to 2 ml	2 to 2.5 ml

How to use the Z-track method

If you're administering iron dextran complex, other irritating drugs, or administering an injection to an elderly patient with decreased muscle mass, you'll vary the standard intramuscular procedure by using the Z-track method. It involves pulling the patient's skin to seal off the needle track after injection, minimizing subcutaneous irritation or discoloration.

You'll inject the drug into the patient's buttock. Never inject more than 5 ml into a single site using this method.

1 After drawing up 0.3 to 0.5 cc of air into the syringe, replace the needle with a sterile one that's 3" (7.5 cm) long. Put on gloves.

Pull the skin laterally away from the intended injection site. This will ensure entry into muscle tissue.

2 After cleaning the site, insert the needle, and inject the drug slowly. When the injection is complete, wait for 10 seconds before withdrawing the needle. This will prevent seepage of the medication from the injection site.

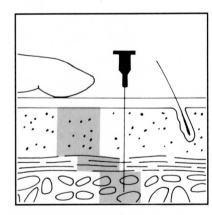

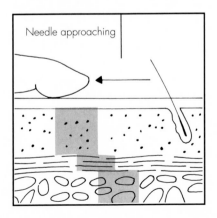

3 After withdrawing the needle, allow the retracted skin to resume its normal position. This will seal off the needle track.

REDUCING THE PAIN OF INTRAMUSCULAR INJECTIONS

You can minimize pain associated with intramuscular injections by following these tips:

• Encourage the patient to relax the muscle. Injections into tense muscles cause more pain and bleeding. To encourage relaxation, give injections into the gluteal muscle while the patient lies face down with toes pointed in, or on his side with the knee and hip of the upper leg flexed and anterior to the lower leg.

• Avoid extra-sensitive areas. When you choose the injection site, roll the muscle mass under your fingers and watch for twitching. This indicates a sensitive "trigger" area. Injections in this area may cause referred pain or a sharp pain as if the nerve were hit.

• Always use a new needle. The point and bevel of the needle can become dulled when they pass through rubber stoppers. Dulled or rough edges cause more friction and pain during injection. Changing the needle also removes another source of pain: irritating medication that adheres to the outside of the needle when you draw the medication out of the vial.

• If you must inject more than 5 ml of solution, divide the solution and inject it at two separate sites, unless the patient's gluteal and vastus lateralis muscles are well developed.

• If the patient has experienced pain or emotional trauma from repeated injections, consider numbing the area before cleaning it by applying ice for several seconds.

Never massage the site or allow the patient to wear a tight fitting garment over the site. Either action could force the medication into the subcutaneous tissue and cause irritation.

To increase the rate of absorption, encourage physical activity, such as walking. For subsequent injections, alternate buttocks.

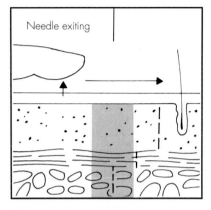

Needle exiting

4 Document your use of the Z-track method.

INFUSION TECHNIQUES

Intravenous Administration

When to give medications intravenously

Administer medications intravenously when you want to:
• immediately treat life-threatening conditions, such as acute epiglottitis or shock.
• quickly achieve and maintain the desired drug level in the patient's bloodstream.
• deliver medications that can't be given by any other route, such as dopamine (Intropin).
• deliver large doses of medication, such as cefoxitin (Mefoxin).
• treat a patient who can't receive medications by any other route, for example, one who's unconscious or who has gastric ulcers.
• avoid damaging subcutaneous or intramuscular layers with potentially harmful drugs, such as levarterenol (Levophed).
• delay drug deactivation by the liver.

Don't administer medication intravenously if:
• an oral form is available and the patient can swallow it.
• the patient has a blood coagulation disorder (unless the medication's needed to treat the coagulation disorder).

I.V. ADMINISTRATION METHODS: HOW THEY DIFFER

METHOD AND PURPOSE	ADVANTAGES	DISADVANTAGES
Direct (I.V. bolus) To deliver drugs rapidly	• Drug takes effect immediately because it's injected directly into bloodstream • Absorption not a factor	• May cause speed shock • More likely to irritate veins • Increases risk of complications, including extravasation, systemic infection, and air embolism
Continuous drip (primary line infusion) To maintain drug delivery at a therapeutic level	• Less irritating than bolus injection • Requires less mixing and hanging than intermittent method • Easy to discontinue	• Can be dangerous if I.V. flow rate isn't carefully monitored • Many drugs don't remain stable for the length of administration • Increases risk of complications, including extravasation, phlebitis, and systemic infection • Drugs administered simultaneously must be compatible • May be difficult to find suitable veins if patient has received previous I.V. therapy
Intermittent To administer drugs mixed with diluent intermittently over time or as a one-time dose, usually via a heparin lock	• Administration time longer than for bolus injection but shorter than for continuous drip therapy • Less likely to cause speed shock than bolus injection • Less irritating to veins than bolus injection • Allows greater mobility	• Frequent use of port increases risk of contamination • Drugs administered simultaneously must be compatible • Increases risk of complications, including extravasation, phlebitis, and systemic infection • Requires flushing injection cap and I.V. catheter with heparin or saline

COMPARING PERIPHERAL VENIPUNCTURE SITES

Venipuncture sites located in the forearm, hand, leg, and foot offer various advantages and disadvantages. The following chart includes some of the major benefits and drawbacks of several common venipuncture sites.

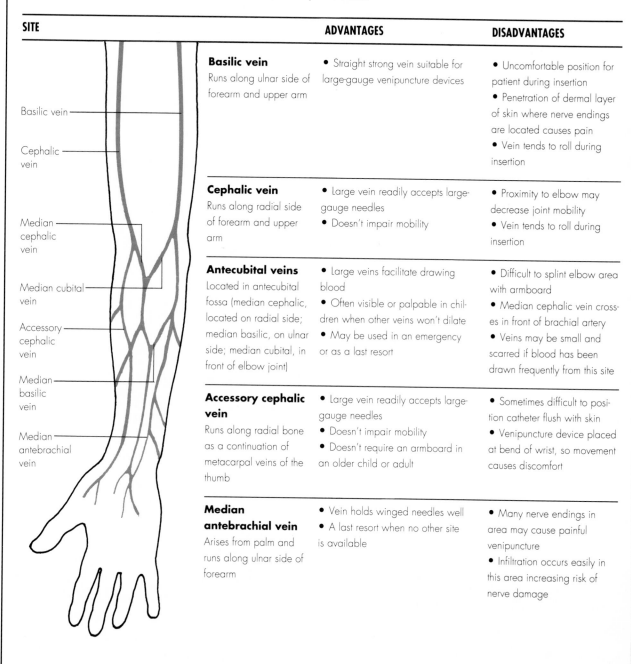

SITE	ADVANTAGES	DISADVANTAGES
Basilic vein Runs along ulnar side of forearm and upper arm	• Straight strong vein suitable for large-gauge venipuncture devices	• Uncomfortable position for patient during insertion • Penetration of dermal layer of skin where nerve endings are located causes pain • Vein tends to roll during insertion
Cephalic vein Runs along radial side of forearm and upper arm	• Large vein readily accepts large-gauge needles • Doesn't impair mobility	• Proximity to elbow may decrease joint mobility • Vein tends to roll during insertion
Antecubital veins Located in antecubital fossa (median cephalic, located on radial side; median basilic, on ulnar side; median cubital, in front of elbow joint)	• Large veins facilitate drawing blood • Often visible or palpable in children when other veins won't dilate • May be used in an emergency or as a last resort	• Difficult to splint elbow area with armboard • Median cephalic vein crosses in front of brachial artery • Veins may be small and scarred if blood has been drawn frequently from this site
Accessory cephalic vein Runs along radial bone as a continuation of metacarpal veins of the thumb	• Large vein readily accepts large-gauge needles • Doesn't impair mobility • Doesn't require an armboard in an older child or adult	• Sometimes difficult to position catheter flush with skin • Venipuncture device placed at bend of wrist, so movement causes discomfort
Median antebrachial vein Arises from palm and runs along ulnar side of forearm	• Vein holds winged needles well • A last resort when no other site is available	• Many nerve endings in area may cause painful venipuncture • Infiltration occurs easily in this area increasing risk of nerve damage

Labels on figure: Basilic vein, Cephalic vein, Median cephalic vein, Median cubital vein, Accessory cephalic vein, Median basilic vein, Median antebrachial vein

continued

COMPARING PERIPHERAL VENIPUNCTURE SITES *continued*

SITE	ADVANTAGES	DISADVANTAGES
Metacarpal veins Located on dorsum of hand; formed by union of digital veins between knuckles	• Easily accessible • Lie flat on back of hand • In adult or large child, bones of hand act as splint	• Wrist mobility decreased unless a short catheter is used • Insertion painful because of the large number of nerve endings in hands • Site becomes phlebitic more easily
Digital veins Run along lateral and dorsal portions of fingers	• May be used for brief therapy • May be used when other sites aren't available	• Fingers must be splinted with a tongue blade, decreasing hand mobility • Uncomfortable for patient • Infiltration occurs easily • Can't be used if metacarpal veins have already been used
Great saphenous vein Located at internal malleolus	• Large vein excellent for venipuncture	• May impair circulation of lower leg • Walking difficult with device in place • Increased risk of deep-vein thrombosis
Dorsal venous network Located on dorsal portion of foot	• Suitable for infants and toddlers	• Vein may be difficult to see or find if edema is present • Walking difficult with device in place • Increased risk of deep-vein thrombosis

Cephalic vein
Basilic vein
Dorsal venous arch
Metacarpal veins
Digital veins

Great saphenous vein
Dorsal venous network

Choosing the venipuncture site

In most cases, the best sites for venipuncture are (in order of preference) the lower arm and hand, the upper arm, and the antecubital fossa. Avoid venipuncture on the patient's legs because it increases the risk of thrombophlebitis and embolism.

Whenever possible, use the distal end of the vein. But first, ask yourself these questions:

• **How long will I.V. therapy last?** For short-term therapy, use the left arm or hand if the patient is right-handed, his right arm or hand if he's left-handed. For long-term therapy, alternate arms and avoid sites over joints.

NURSING TIP   If a patient will require long-term I.V. therapy, get maximum use from his arm veins by starting the therapy in a hand vein, then switching to sites farther up his arm, as necessary.

• **What kind of I.V. solution's been ordered?**

For infusions that are highly acidic, alkaline, or hypertonic, use a large vein to adequately dilute the infusion. A small peripheral vein may become irritated. Rapid infusions also require larger veins.

• **What size needle or cannula are you using?**

If the solution's highly viscous, you'll need a large-bore needle or cannula. Then, choose a vein that's big enough to accommodate it.

• **Is the vein full, soft, and unobstructed?**

Palpate the patient's veins to find one that's not crooked, hardened, scarred, or inflamed. If you must perform venipuncture on a leg, avoid using a varicose vein. However, if you must use one, elevate the patient's leg during the infusion.

If the patient's veins are neither visible nor palpable, you may find a fiberoptic illuminator helpful (see *Locating hard-to-find veins*, page 84). To use it, turn off the room lights, and attach the illuminator to the patient's limb. His limb will appear red and the veins black.

• **Does the patient have any specific problems or injuries that require special consideration?**

Avoid using veins in irritated, infected, or injured areas because the added stress of venipuncture may cause complications. If the patient has had a radical mastectomy or a dialysis fistula, don't start an I.V. in the arm on that side of the body.

• **How old is the patient?**

If the patient's an adolescent or an adult, the hand or lower arm will probably provide the best site. If the patient is an infant, the useable sites are the hands, feet, ankles, inner aspect of the wrists, and the antecubital area. The scalp veins may offer easier insertion sites for infants under age 6 months; however, you must palpate the artery.

How to spike and prime I.V. solutions

When preparing to place an I.V. line, you must spike the container and run I.V. fluid through the tubing to expel all the air. This simple but important process is called spiking and priming.

Wash your hands thoroughly and gather your equipment: the prescribed I.V. solution and an administration set. Select vented I.V. tubing for a solution in a nonvented bottle; nonvented tubing for a solution in a bag or vented bottle.

Spiking a nonvented bottle

1 Remove the bottle's metal cap and inner disk, if present. Place the bottle on a stable surface, and wipe the rubber stopper with alcohol.

2 Remove the cap from the administration set spike, and push the spike through the center of the bottle's rubber stopper. Avoid twisting or angling the spike to prevent pieces of the stopper from breaking off and falling into the solution.

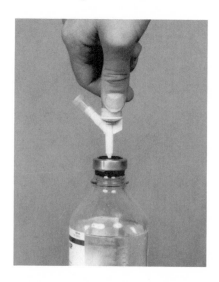

3 Invert the bottle. If its vacuum is intact, you'll hear a hissing sound and see air bubbles rise (this may not occur if you've added medication). If it is not intact, discard the bottle.

4 Hang the bottle on the I.V. pole, and squeeze the drip chamber until it is half full.

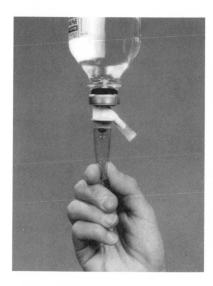

Spiking a vented bottle

1 Remove the bottle's metal cap and latex diaphragm to release the vacuum as shown. If the vacuum is not intact, discard the bottle. Place the bottle on a stable surface, and wipe the rubber stopper with alcohol.

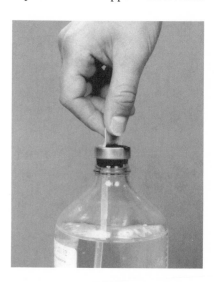

GUIDE TO NEEDLE AND CATHETER GAUGES

How do you know which gauge needle and catheter to use for your patient? The answer depends on your patient's age and condition and on the type of infusion he's receiving. The following chart lists the uses and nursing considerations for the various gauges.

GAUGE	USES	NURSING CONSIDERATIONS
16	• Adolescents and adults • Major surgery • Trauma • Infusion of large volumes of fluids	• Painful insertion • Requires large vein
18	• Older children, adolescents, and adults • Administration of blood and blood components and other viscous infusions	• Painful insertion • Requires large vein
20	• Children, adolescents, and adults • Suitable for most I.V. infusions	• Commonly used
22	• Infants, toddlers, children, adolescents, and adults (especially elderly patients) • Suitable for most I.V. infusions	• Easier to insert in small, thin, fragile veins • Slower flow rates must be maintained • More difficult to insert into tough skin
24, 26	• Neonates, infants, toddlers, school-age children, adolescents, and adults (especially elderly patients) • Suitable for most infusions, but flow rates are slower	• For extremely small veins, such as small veins of fingers or veins of inner arms in elderly patients • May be difficult to insert into tough skin

2 Remove the protective cap from the administration set spike, and push the spike through the insertion port next to the air vent tube opening.

3 Hang the bottle on the I.V. pole, and squeeze the drip chamber until it is half full.

Spiking a bag

1 Place the bag on a flat, stable surface or hang it on an I.V. pole. Then, remove the protective cap or tear tab from the tubing insertion port, and wipe the port with an alcohol pad.

2 Remove the protective cap from the administration set spike.

3 Holding the port carefully and firmly with one hand, quickly insert the spike with your other hand as shown.

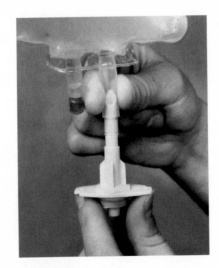

4 Hang the bag about 36" (90 cm) above the selected venipuncture site and squeeze the drip chamber until it is half full.

Priming the I.V. tubing

1 If desired, attach a filter to the other end of the I.V. tubing, and follow the manufacturer's instructions for filling and priming.

2 If you're not using a filter, remove the protective cap in the tubing. Then, while maintaining the sterility of the tubing's end, hold it over a wastebasket or sink, and open the flow clamp as shown.

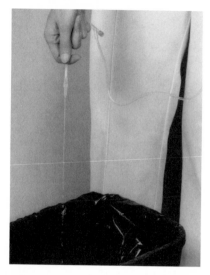

3 Leave the clamp open until I.V. solution flows through the entire length of tubing, forcing out all air. Invert all Y injection sites and backcheck valves, and tap them, if necessary, to fill them with solution.

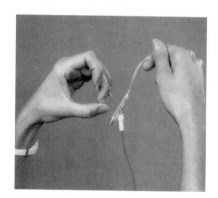

4 Close the clamp and replace the protective cover. Then, loop the tubing over the I.V. pole.

5 Label the container with the patient's name and room number, the date and time, the container number, the ordered duration of infusion, and your initials. Place an

I.V. time tape or a strip of adhesive tape on the bottle and mark the amount of fluid to be infused hourly.

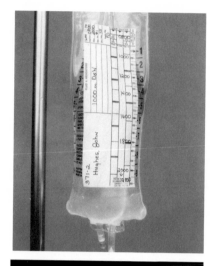

How to prime a filter

As you begin, remember that you must always use aseptic technique to connect one part of a delivery system to another. Then, once you've minimized the risk of contamination, proceed as follows.

1 Remove the caps from the administration set and the filter. Fit the tubing's male adapter into the filter's female connector. Twist it firmly to make a snug connection.

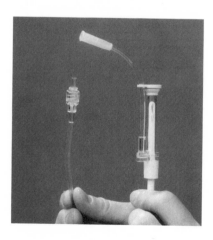

2 Hold the filter so the male-female joint is pointed down, as shown. Then, open all the clamps on the line to prime the tubing and the filter. Tap the filter housing to dislodge air bubbles. When the filter is primed, close the roller clamp. Now you're ready to perform venipuncture.

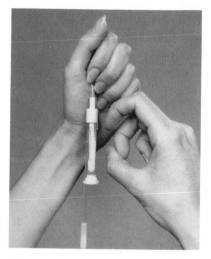

3 If the filter is built into the line, like the one shown here, prime it in the same way.

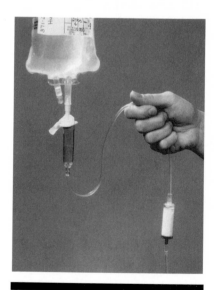

GUIDELINES FOR USING IN-LINE I.V. FILTERS

An in-line I.V. filter, such as the 0.22-micron model, removes pathogens and particles from I.V. solutions, helping to reduce the risk of infusion phlebitis. Because installing a filter is costly, cumbersome, and time consuming, it is not routinely used. Consequently, many institutions require use of a filter only for administration of an admixture. If you're unsure whether or not to use a filter, follow these guidelines.

Use an in-line I.V. filter:

• for any infusion to an immunodeficient patient.
• for intravenous total parenteral nutrition.
• when using additives comprising many separate particles, such as antibiotics requiring reconstitution, or when administering several additives.
• when using rubber injection sites or plastic diaphragms frequently.
• when phlebitis is likely .
   Change in-line I.V. filters at least every 24 hours. If you don't, bacteria trapped in the filter release endotoxin, a pyrogen small enough to pass through the filter into the bloodstream.

Avoid using an in-line filter:

• when administering solutions with large particles that will clog the filter and stop I.V. flow, for example, blood and its components, suspensions such as amphotericin B (Fungizone), emulsions such as Liposyn, and high–molecular-volume plasma expanders such as dextran (Gentran).
• when administering a small dosage of a drug (5 mg or less) because the filter may absorb it.

How to add and prime a filter

Filters range in size from 0.22 micron (the most common) to 170 microns. Some filters are built into the line, such as the one shown in How to Prime a Filter; others need to be added. Filter needles, such as the one shown here, may be used if drugs are not prepared by the pharmacist. They are most commonly used for mixing lyophilized (powdered) drugs and drugs in glass ampules.

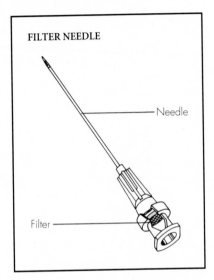

FILTER NEEDLE

Needle

Filter

If a filter needle is not available, you can make one by following these simple steps:

1   Pull back the tabs on the add-a-filter and the needle packages, following the manufacturer's directions.

2   Attach the filter needle to the syringe.

3   Draw up the medication.

Discard the filter needle and replace it with a regular needle after you've drawn up the medication.

Performing Venipuncture

Before venipuncture, you need to dilate the vein, prepare the venipuncture site, stabilize the vein, and then insert the venipuncture device. After the infusion is started, you can complete the I.V. placement by securing the device with tape or a transparent dressing.

How to dilate a vein

To dilate or distend a vein effectively, you need to use a tourniquet, which traps blood in the veins by applying enough pressure to impede venous flow. A properly distended vein should appear and feel round, firm, and fully filled with blood and should rebound when compressed. Because the amount of trapped blood depends on arterial circulation, a patient who's hypotensive, very cold, or experiencing vasomotor changes (such as septic shock) may have inadequate filling of the peripheral blood vessels.

Before applying the tourniquet, place the patient's arm in a dependent position to increase capillary fill of the lower arms and hands. If his skin is cold, warm it by rubbing and stroking his arm or covering the entire arm with warm packs for 5 to 10 minutes. As soon as you remove the warm packs, apply the tourniquet and perform the venipuncture.

The ideal tourniquet can be tied easily, doesn't roll into a thin band, stays relatively flat, and is easy to release. Many types are available. Some have a catch mechanism to anchor them. Others have a wide, flat rubber band that's secured with Velcro. The most common type is a soft rubber tourniquet about 2" (5.1 cm) wide. To tie it, follow these steps.

1 Place the tourniquet under the patient's arm, about 6" (15.2 cm) above the intended venipuncture site (for example, on the midlower arm for hand and arm veins). Position the arm on the middle of the tourniquet.

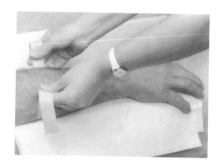

2 Bring the ends of the tourniquet together and place one on top of the other.

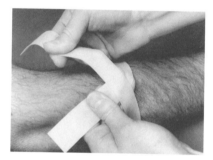

3 Holding one end on top of the other, lift and stretch the tourniquet and tuck the top tail under the bottom tail. Don't allow the tourniquet to loosen.

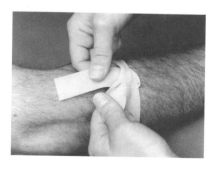

4 Tie the tourniquet smoothly and snugly, being careful not to pinch the patient's skin or pull his arm hair. Leave the tourniquet in place no longer than 2 minutes. If you can't find a suitable vein and prepare the venipuncture site within this time, release the tourniquet for a few minutes. Then reapply it and continue the procedure. You may need to apply the tourniquet, find the vein, remove the tourniquet, prepare the site, and then reapply the tourniquet for the venipuncture.

5 Keep the tourniquet as flat as possible. It should be snug but not uncomfortably tight. If it's too tight, it'll impede arterial as well as venous blood flow. Check the patient's radial pulse. If you can't feel it, the tourniquet is too tight and must be loosened. Also loosen and reapply the tourniquet if the patient complains of severe tightness.

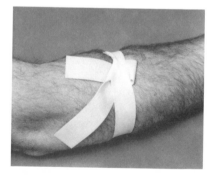

6 Once you've applied the tourniquet, have the patient open and close his fist tightly four to six times.

Flick the skin over the vein with one or two sharp snaps of your fore-

LOCATING HARD-TO-FIND VEINS

New tools are available to help locate hard-to-find veins. The Landry Vein Light (LVL), a small transilluminating instrument, uses a bright light from two adjustable fiber-optic arms to help visualize deeply concealed peripheral veins.

This instrument works best in a dimly lit room. With the LVL on its brightest setting, the nurse scans the limb below the tourniquet for a vein. The vein will appear as a dark line between the fiberoptic arms. Of course, it will take practice to learn to place a needle correctly in the dim lighting the LVL requires.

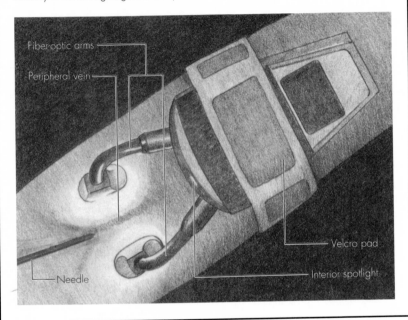

Fiber-optic arms

Peripheral vein

Needle

Velcro pad

Interior spotlight

finger. This is less traumatic than slapping the skin, yet it achieves the same effect of distending the vein.

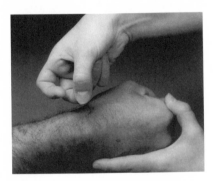

7 Rub or stroke the skin upward toward the tourniquet. If the vein still feels small and soft, release the

tourniquet. Reapply it a little tighter and closer to the venipuncture site than before.

8 If the vein still isn't well distended, remove the tourniquet, apply a warm pack for 5 minutes and reapply the tourniquet. This is especially helpful if the patient's skin is cool.

Remember that a tourniquet applied too tightly or kept in place too long may cause increased bruising, especially in elderly patients whose veins are fragile. Release the tourniquet as soon as you've placed the venipuncture device into the vein. You'll know the device is in the vein when you see blood in the venipuncture device's flashback chamber.

NURSING TIP Current research suggests that fist clenching during phlebotomy could falsely elevate serum potassium levels.

How to prepare the venipuncture site

Before performing the venipuncture you'll need to clean the site.

1 Place an absorbent pad under the venipuncture site, then put on gloves. Clip the hair over the insertion site.

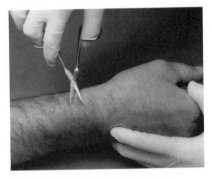

2 Clean the skin with a thin coat of a solution such as povidone iodine (Betadine), tincture of iodine, or 70% alcohol. Wipe the skin, starting at the center of the insertion site and moving outward with a circular motion. To reduce the risk of contamination, use a swab stick, as shown, or swab ampule rather than a pad. Don't go over an area you've already cleaned. Allow the solution to dry (this takes 30 to 60 seconds).

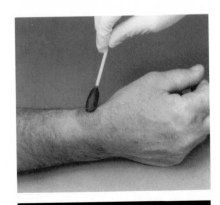

How to use a steel winged needle

Commonly called butterfly needles, steel winged needles have no hub, lie flat on the skin, and make taping easy. These devices range in size from 16G to 27G and are about ¾" (1.9 cm) long. They're short, thin walled, and extremely sharp. Their single-needle design makes them the easiest device to insert. But because they have a steel needle instead of a plastic catheter, the risk of infiltration during patient movement is greater. Originally designed for pediatric and geriatric use, steel winged needles should be used when a patient is in stable condition, has adequate veins, and requires I.V. fluids or medications for only a short time. It's also ideal for single I.V. push injections, such as chemotherapy.

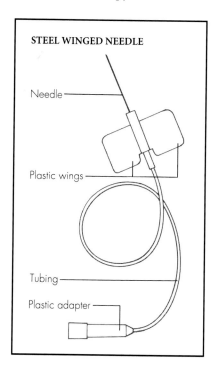

STEEL WINGED NEEDLE

Needle

Plastic wings

Tubing

Plastic adapter

If you've already gathered the necessary equipment, washed your hands, put on gloves, and explained venipuncture to the patient, you're ready to insert the steel winged needle into his vein.

1 Spike the fluid container and attach the tubing adapter to the needle connector, as shown.

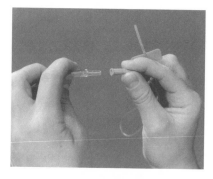

Flush both the tubing and the needle with fluid to remove air. Clamp the tube to stop fluid flow, and recap the needle to maintain sterility.

2 Select a vein and prepare the venipuncture site.

Next, remove the needle cap. Point the needle in the direction of the blood flow and hold it at a 45-degree angle above the skin, with the bevel facing up. Now you're ready to insert the needle into the vein, using what's commonly called the indirect method of venipuncture.

Pinch the wings together tightly, as shown. Keeping your hand steady, pierce the patient's skin at a point slightly to one side of the vein, about ½" (1.3 cm) below the spot where you plan to puncture the vein wall.

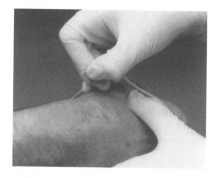

3 Decrease the needle angle until the needle's almost level with the skin surface, and direct it toward the vein

you've selected. You'll feel very little resistance as the needle goes through subcutaneous tissue; you'll feel considerably more resistance when you reach the vein.

Proceeding carefully, attempt to puncture the vein with the needle. To confirm that you've punctured the vein, watch for blood backflow in the tubing (for more details, see How to Check Needle Placement and Flow Rate, page 86).

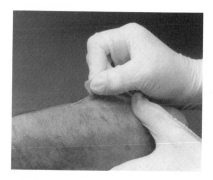

4 Continue to advance the needle until it's well within the vein. By exerting a gentle, lifting pressure during insertion, you can keep the needle from piercing the opposite wall of the vein.

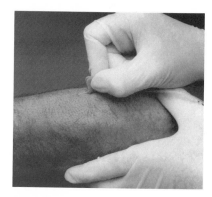

5 To begin the infusion, remove the tourniquet from the patient's arm, open the flow clamp in the tubing, and check for free flow. Then, partially close the clamp until you've securely taped the needle and tubing.

STABILIZING A VEIN FOR VENIPUNCTURE

To help ensure successful venipuncture, you need to stabilize the patient's vein by stretching the skin and holding it taut. The stretching technique you'll use varies with different venipuncture sites. To stabilize the cephalic vein above the wrist, have the patient make a tight fist. Then stretch his fist laterally downward and immobilize the skin with the thumb of your other hand, as shown.

Stabilizing techniques for other sites are described below.

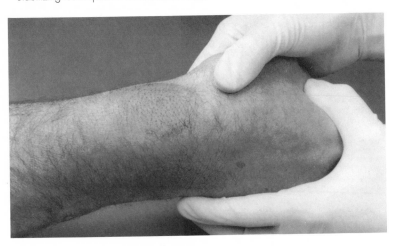

SITE	TECHNIQUE
Hand veins	Stretch the patient's hand and wrist downward and hold your thumb over his fingers.
Basilic vein at outer arm	Have the patient make a tight fist and flex his elbow. Stand behind the flexed arm, retract the skin away from the site, and anchor the vein with your thumb. Or, rotate the patient's extended lower arm inward and approach the vein from behind the arm (may be difficult for the patient to maintain).
Inner aspect of wrist	Extend the patient's open hand backward from the wrist. Anchor the vein with your thumb below the insertion site.
Inner arm	Extend the patient's closed fist backward from the wrist. Anchor the vein with your thumb above the wrist.
Antecubital fossa	Have the patient form a tight fist and extend his arm completely. Anchor the skin with your thumb about 2" or 3" (5.1 or 7.6 cm) below the antecubital fossa.
Saphenous vein of ankle	Extend the patient's foot downward and inward. Anchor the vein with your thumb about 2" or 3" below the ankle.
Dorsum of foot	Pull the patient's foot downward. Anchor the vein with your thumb about 2" to 3" below the vein (usually near the toes).

How to check needle placement and flow rate

The following tips will help you confirm needle placement and maintain the prescribed flow rate.

1 The best way to tell if you've entered the vein is by checking for blood backflow. Lower the I.V. container below the venipuncture site. Bend the tubing at a point several inches away from the needle or cannula and then release it. If the needle is properly placed in the vein, gravity usually pulls blood into the tubing.

2 If the flow rate is sluggish when you begin the infusion, slightly advance the needle or cannula, and check the flow rate again. You may also get backflow when the needle or cannula has passed through the vein and out the opposite wall, but it will be minimal. If you try for backflow after a moment, you won't get any.

3 Another cause of sluggish flow is that the needle or catheter may be jammed against the vein wall. Try pulling it back slightly, about ⅛" (0.6 cm) as shown. You may also try rotating a catheter gently, but don't manipulate a winged-tip needle this way. If you do, the needle's bevel may injure the vein, triggering infiltration or thrombophlebitis.

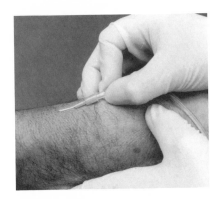

4 Sometimes a clot in the needle or catheter blocks the infusion. Close the flow clamp, and try aspirating the clot with a syringe on the catheter hub. (Take care not to contaminate the hub or the tubing.) If that doesn't work, restart the I.V. in another vein.

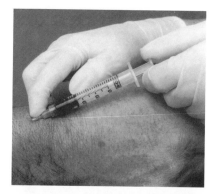

Never try irrigating a clogged I.V. with a syringe and solution. You'll increase the chance of infection and risk propelling the clot into the bloodstream.

5 In some cases, you can restore flow by changing the angle of the needle or catheter. To do this, elevate it slightly with a sterile cotton ball, a 2" × 2" gauze pad, or a tongue blade.

6 To lower a catheter slightly, put a sterile cotton ball, a 2" × 2" gauze pad, or a tongue blade over it, and secure it with tape.

NURSING TIP The needle or catheter angle may be affected by patient movement. If you find that the drip rate varies when the patient moves his arm, apply a splint to stabilize the needle or catheter (see How to Apply Splints and Restraints, pages 91 and 92). Never tape so tightly that blood flow's impeded.

How to insert an over-the-needle catheter

An over-the-needle catheter (ONC) is useful for long-term therapy for the active or agitated patient.

An ONC is less likely to puncture a vein than a needle, is more comfortable for the patient once it's in place, contains radiopaque thread for easy location, and some units come with a syringe attached that permits easy check of blood return and prevents air from entering the vessel on insertion. However, an ONC is more difficult to insert than other devices.

The initial steps for inserting an ONC are the same as for inserting a

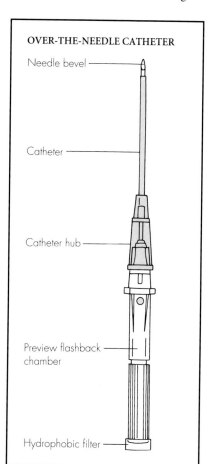

OVER-THE-NEEDLE CATHETER

Needle bevel

Catheter

Catheter hub

Preview flashback chamber

Hydrophobic filter

winged-tip needle (see page 85). Then, follow the same procedure to place the ONC securely in the vein. After you've checked for blood backflow, follow these steps to complete

the procedure. (See page 88 for a discussion of the PROTECTIV catheter, a device that decreases the risk of needle-stick accidents.)

1 Have a 4" × 4" sterile gauze pad ready to slip under the hub as soon as the cannula is in place. (If you prefer, use a skin prep swab instead.) This provides a firm, sterile field for the connection point and protects the hub and adapter from touch contamination. It will also catch any blood that spills when you withdraw the needle. If it becomes soiled, remove it after you connect the hub and adapter.

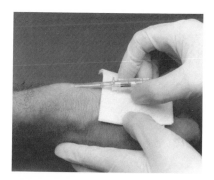

2 Hold the needle hub firmly in place with your thumb and forefinger. Now, advance the cannula another ¼" (0.6 cm) to make sure it's in the vein properly. Because the catheter's slightly shorter than the needle, blood backflow sometimes occurs when the needle alone is in the vein. The extra ¼" advancement ensures that the cannula's placed in the vein lumen.

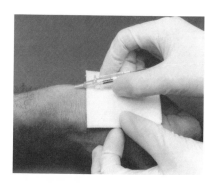

NOTE If you feel any resistance, don't force the catheter. Instead, withdraw the needle and catheter together. If you try to withdraw the catheter first, you may cut it on the needle's sharp bevel, creating a catheter embolus. Attempt venipuncture again at another site.

3 When you're sure the cannula's placed correctly, release the tourniquet and withdraw the needle. If the needle sticks inside the catheter, grasp the catheter hub firmly, and rotate the needle to loosen it.

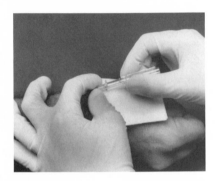

4 As you remove the needle, you may want to press lightly on the skin over the catheter tip to prevent bleeding, as shown.

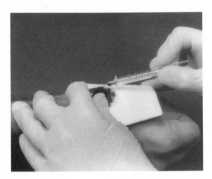

5 Connect the adapter of the administration set to the catheter hub. When you've completed the connection, let the I.V. fluid flow freely for a few seconds to assure proper placement of the catheter.

Apply antimicrobial ointment to the I.V. site if policy requires. Then, set a slow flow rate until you finish dressing and taping the site (see How to Tape Venipuncture Devices).

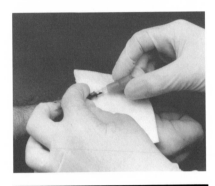

How to use a PROTECTIV catheter

The PROTECTIV catheter is a disposable device that decreases the risk of needle-stick accidents.

As the nurse slides the catheter off the needle, a protective guard glides into place over the needle. The contaminated needle can then be discarded safely.

1 Insert the I.V. catheter. Then, with your forefinger, advance the push-off tab to begin threading the catheter.

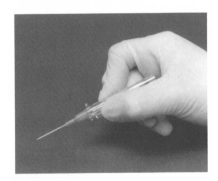

2 Slide the catheter off the introducer needle and move the protective guard over the needle. A "click" signals that the needle is locked in place.

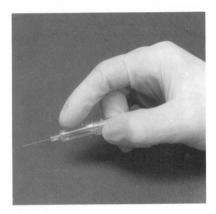

3 Remove the covered, locked needle from the catheter hub for safe disposal.

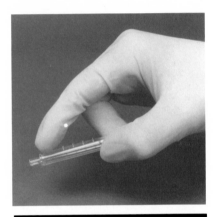

How to secure the venipuncture device

After the infusion begins, you must secure the venipuncture device at the insertion site with tape or a transparent semipermeable dressing. If necessary, trim excess hair from the site before you apply the tape to improve visibility of the veins and the site, and to reduce pain when the tape is removed

1 If policy requires, place a small amount of antiseptic ointment directly over the insertion site. (This ointment should be applied daily.)

INSIDE-THE-NEEDLE CATHETER

An inside-the-needle catheter (INC) differs from the over-the-needle catheter primarily in the way the cannula is housed and advanced. Because the cannula travels inside the introducer needle, it creates a larger puncture site. Such catheters are most often used for administering drugs or solutions that could cause extravasation if infiltration occurs, or when venous access is poor. An INC is useful for long-term therapy for the active or agitated patient and for central venous insertion.

An INC is less likely to puncture a vein than a needle, is more comfortable for the patient once it's in place, is available in many lengths, and most contain radiopaque thread for easy location.

However, an INC may leak at the site, especially in elderly patients, and if the needle guard is not used, the catheter may be severed and enter the circulation, creating an embolus.

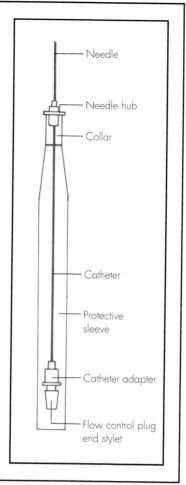

- Needle
- Needle hub
- Collar
- Catheter
- Protective sleeve
- Catheter adapter
- Flow control plug end stylet

4 Remove the old dressing every 1 to 2 days or as policy requires, and clean the insertion site with povidone-iodine solution (Betadine). As always, start at the center and wipe toward the periphery using a circular motion. If residue remains on the skin, clean it with alcohol. Allow the skin to dry, then apply tape in the usual manner.

After applying tape or a dressing, be sure to label it as shown with the date and time of I.V. insertion, the name and gauge of the venipuncture device, and your initials.

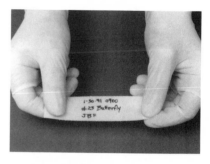

If the patient's arm must be immobilized during infusion, you may need to apply an armboard (see How to Apply Splints and Restraints, page 91). Remember to document your interventions carefully after you've performed the venipuncture.

How to tape venipuncture devices

If you'll be using tape to secure the venipuncture device to the insertion site, use one of the three basic methods described below.

Chevron method

1 Cover the venipuncture site with an adhesive strip or a 2" × 2" sterile gauze pad. Then cut a long strip of ½" (1.3 cm) tape. Place it, sticky side

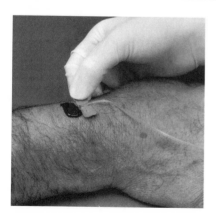

2 Apply an adhesive bandage or a sterile 2" × 2" gauze pad directly over the insertion site.

3 Use one of the taping methods covered in How to Tape Venipuncture Devices. Remember to use as little tape as possible and don't let the tape ends meet. This reduces the risk of a tourniquet effect should infiltration occur. Don't allow the tape to cover the patient's skin beyond the device's tip. This could obscure swelling and redness. If the patient has had a previous allergic reaction to tape, use a hypoallergenic tape (preferably one that's lightweight and easy to remove). Usually, paper tape isn't satisfactory for I.V. sites because it shreds and is difficult to remove.

up, under the needle, parallel to the short strip of tape or gauze pad.

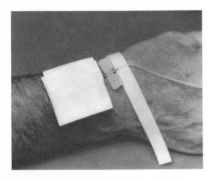

2 Cross the ends of the tape over the needle so that the tape sticks to the patient's skin.

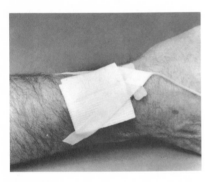

3 Apply a piece of 1" (2.5 cm) tape across the two wings of the chevron.

Loop the tubing and secure it with another piece of 1" tape. On the tape, write the date and time of insertion, the type and gauge of the needle, and your initials.

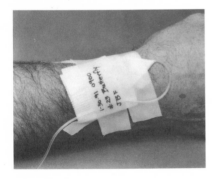

U method

1 Cover the venipuncture site with an adhesive strip or a 2" × 2" sterile gauze pad. Then cut three strips of ½" tape. With the sticky side up, place one strip under the tubing as shown for the chevron method.

2 Bring each side of the tape up, folding it over the wings of the needle, as shown. Press it down, parallel to the tubing. Apply a piece of ½" tape at each end of the gauze pad.

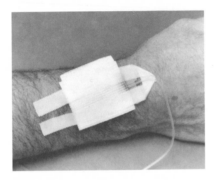

3 Loop the tubing and secure it with a piece of 1" tape. On the tape, write the date and time of insertion, the type and gauge of the needle or catheter, and your initials.

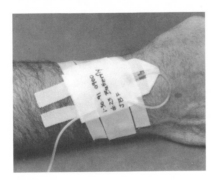

H method

1 Cover the venipuncture site with an adhesive strip or a 2" × 2" gauze pad. Then cut three strips of 1" tape.

2 Place one strip of tape over each wing, keeping the tape parallel to the needle.

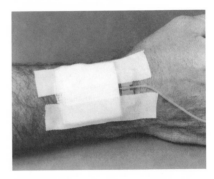

3 Place the other strip of tape perpendicular to the first two. Put it either directly on top of the wings or just below the wings, directly on top of the tubing. On the last piece of tape, write the date and time of insertion, the type and gauge of the needle or catheter, and your initials.

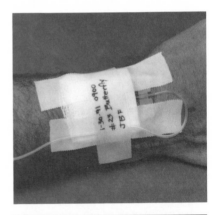

How to apply a transparent semipermeable dressing

Because it helps to prevent infection, many institutions now use a transparent semipermeable dressing on an I.V. insertion site instead of tape. This dressing allows air to pass through it, but it's impervious to microorganisms. If the dressing remains intact, daily changes aren't necessary. Its other advantages include fewer skin reactions and a clearly visible insertion site helpful in detecting the early signs of phlebitis and swelling. The waterproof tape protects the site from contamination should it become wet and it adheres well to the skin, with less risk of accidental dislodgment of the device.

1 Make sure the insertion site is clean and dry.

2 Place the dressing directly over the insertion site and the hub, as shown. Cover as little tubing as possible. Don't stretch the dressing because doing so may cause itching.

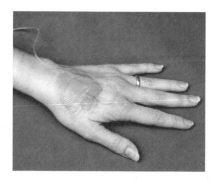

3 Tuck the dressing around and under the catheter hub to make the site occlusive to microorganisms.

4 To remove the dressing, stabilize the needle hub with your nondominant hand, then grasp one corner of the dressing with your dominant hand and lift and stretch the dressing.

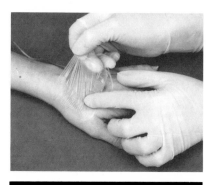

PROTECTING A SCALP VEIN SITE

To protect a venipuncture site on an infant's scalp, use a commercially available protective device as shown. Cover the edges of the device with tape and place it over the needle so the tubing extends through the tunnel. Secure the device with strips of tape.

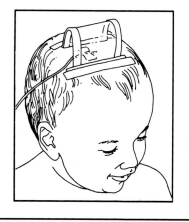

How to apply splints and restraints

When the venipuncture site's at a joint and flexion may impede flow of I.V. fluids or if your patient's restless and extravasation is a concern, consider applying a splint to stabilize the needle or catheter. A confused or combative patient may need the added protection of restraints. However, don't apply restraints without a doctor's order.

1 To determine if your patient needs an armboard, move his limb through its full range of motion while watching the I.V. flow rate. If the flow stops during movement, you'll need to apply an armboard.

Which is better, a long or short splint? A short splint is adequate

when the site's on the hand or lower arm. You'll need a long one to protect a site in the antecubital fossa. Most splints are disposable and covered with plastic. For the patient's comfort, pad the splint with a washcloth or another soft material.

Choose a splint that's long enough to prevent flexion and extension at the tip of the device. Then, position the arm palm down to keep the body properly aligned and to prevent injury to the upper arm's nerves and muscles. Make sure the hand is supported by the end of the splint, as shown.

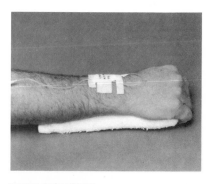

NURSING TIP In a pinch, you can fashion a splint from a rolled towel, a tissue box, or an I.V. tubing box. Because such improvisations won't hold up for an active patient, replace them with a splint as soon as possible.

2 To ensure free blood circulation and ease the eventual removal of the splint, you'll want to face, or backstrap, the adhesive securing the splint as shown. To do this, first tear two strips of tape of equal width, one the diameter of the patient's arm and the other twice that length. Then, put the shorter piece in the center of the long one, with the sticky sides together.

Prepare at least three of these faced tape strips if you're using a long splint, two to secure a short one.

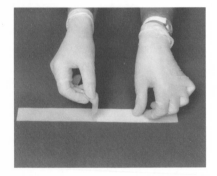

Now, wrap the tape around the arm and splint, keeping the faced part of the tape against the patient's arm and the sticky part against the splint. Tape securely enough to immobilize the arm, but take care not to impede circulation.

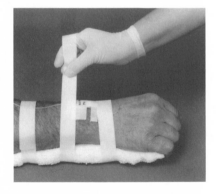

Don't tape over the venipuncture site. This way, you can easily remove the dressing to observe the site.

If the splint will be in place for a long time, encourage the patient to exercise his hand periodically by squeezing a rubber ball or gauze roll.

NURSING TIP As an alternative to taping the splint in the above manner, wrap gauze around both the splint and the arm or use stretch netting.

3 If your patient's *very* restless and the doctor's ordered restraints, remember that the patient may be upset by the idea that he needs to be restrained. Tactfully explain how restraints will help keep his I.V. line in place. Avoid using a judgmental tone; don't give the impression you're punishing him.

If the venipuncture site's on the hand or forearm, just slip the gauze under the patient's arm and around the splint. If you apply a restraint without splinting the arm, don't tie the gauze in such a way that the catheter presses down on the vein. This will irritate the vein and increase the risk of phlebitis.

If the patient's a child or a confused adult, keep the flow clamp out of his reach. Running a strip of tape beneath the clamp will prevent him from pulling it down.

Now, tie the other end of the restraint to the bed frame, toward the foot of the bed.

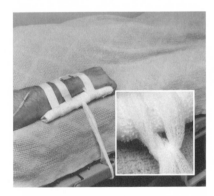

If both arms are restrained, keep the restraints short enough to keep the arms apart. But don't make them so short that the patient can't move at all. If the patient's turned on his side, adjust the restraints so his arms don't touch. Use a pillow to keep his arms apart.

For safety's sake, don't tie the restraint to the bed's side rail. Make sure the knot's out of the patient's reach once the bed rail's raised. Remember, a patient who needs restraints must never be left unattended with the bed rails down.

NURSING TIP For some patients you may need only a 2" (5.1 cm) stockinette or stretch netting to protect the site. In such cases, cut a hole for the thumb, and bring the stockinette up over the I.V. site. Roll it back to inspect the site.

How to make a mummy restraint

A mummy restraint is a temporary total body restraint used to immobilize an infant or young child during a procedure such as venipuncture.

1 Lay the infant in the center of a draw sheet or towel.

2 Fold the right side of the restraint over the infant's arm and tuck the edge under the infant's trunk.

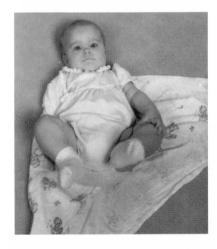

3 Fold the left side of the restraint over the infant's left arm and tuck the edge under the left side of the trunk.

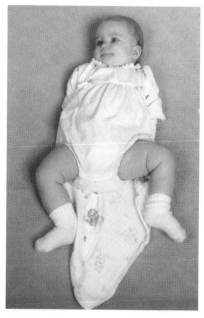

4 To immobilize the legs, lay another draw sheet over the infant and tuck under each side. This secures the child firmly without creating pressure that could constrict respirations.

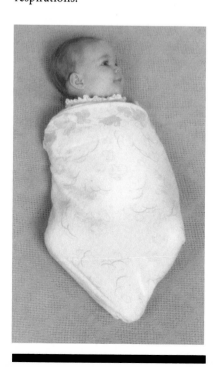

DOCUMENTING VENIPUNCTURE

When you start an I.V. line, be sure to document the following:
- date and time of venipuncture
- lot number of the solution container (if policy requires)
- type and amount of solution
- name and dosage of additives in the solution
- type of venipuncture device used, including length and gauge
- venipuncture site
- number of insertion attempts (if more than one)
- flow rate
- adverse reactions and actions taken to correct them
- patient teaching and evidence of patient understanding
- name of the person initiating the infusion
- whether a splint or restraints were used.

Treating extravasation

Extravasation (the infiltration of a drug into surrounding tissue) can result from a punctured vein or from leakage around a venipuncture site. Extravasation of vesicant (blistering) drugs or fluids often causes severe local tissue damage and carries the risk of prolonged healing, infection, multiple debridements, cosmetic disfigurement, loss of function, and amputation.

Extravasation of vesicant drugs calls for emergency treatment as follows:
- Stop the I.V. flow and remove the I.V. line, unless you need the needle to infiltrate the antidote.
- Estimate the amount of extravasated solution and notify the doctor.
- Instill the appropriate antidote according to institution policy.
- Elevate the extremity.

- Record the extravasation site, the patient's symptoms, the estimated amount of infiltrated solution, and treatment provided. Also record the time you notified the doctor and his name. Continue documenting the site's appearance and associated symptoms.
- Apply ice packs or warm compresses to the affected area, according to policy.
- If skin breakdown occurs, apply silver sulfadiazine cream and gauze dressings or wet-to-dry povidone-iodine dressings, as ordered.

How to discontinue an I.V.

1 Wash your hands thoroughly and put on gloves. Then, stop the patient's I.V. fluid flow completely by closing off the flow clamp. Carefully remove the tape and dressing, taking care not to disturb the needle or catheter.

2 Hold a 2" × 2" sterile gauze pad just above the site as shown. Then, quickly withdraw the needle or catheter, pulling straight back to avoid tearing the vein. Immediately apply pressure to the site with a 2" × 2" sterile gauze pad, and hold it against the site until the bleeding has stopped. This prevents blood from oozing out of the vein and causing a hematoma.

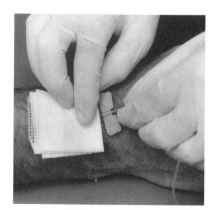

Finally, tape down the pad and leave it in place for 10 minutes. Don't use an adhesive bandage strip, because it won't exert enough pressure to stop the bleeding. Don't apply alcohol; it will irritate the wound and inhibit clotting.

Have the patient hold the arm upward for 5 minutes. After 10 minutes, the pressure dressing may be replaced with a small adhesive bandage. Instruct the patient to have the bandage removed after 8 hours.

Infusing I.V. Solution

How to calculate the flow rate

1 To calculate the correct flow rate, answer these questions:
• How much solution did the doctor order?
• How much time is allowed for delivery?

2 Take the amount of solution to be administered and divide it by the delivery time

$$\frac{1000 \text{ ml}}{8 \text{ hours}} = 125 \text{ ml/hour}$$

3 Decide which type of drip system you're using. If you're delivering a lot of fluid in a short time, use a macrodrip system. The macrodrip, depending on the manufacturer, takes 10, 15, or 20 gtt to deliver 1 ml. If you're delivering a small amount of fluid over a long time, use a microdrip system. The microdrip takes 60 gtt to deliver 1 ml.

Insert your answers into this formula:

$$\frac{\text{drops/ml}}{60 \text{ minutes}} \times \frac{\text{amount of fluid/hour}}{1} = \text{drops/minute}$$

If you're using a macrodrip system, your equation will look like one of these:

$$\frac{10}{60} \times \frac{125}{1} = \frac{125}{6} = 21 \text{ gtt/minute}$$

$$\frac{15}{60} \times \frac{125}{1} = \frac{125}{4} = 31 \text{ gtt/minute}$$

$$\frac{20}{60} \times \frac{125}{1} = \frac{125}{3} = 41 \text{ gtt/minute}$$

If you're using a microdrip system, your equation will look like this:

$$\frac{60}{60} \times \frac{125}{1} = 125 \text{ gtt/minute}$$

4 After you've determined the rate, setting the flow is easy. When you've established your I.V. line, slowly open the clamp to start fluid dripping into the drip chamber. Hold your watch close to the chamber, and time the drips for 1 minute as shown. Open or close the clamp as needed to adjust the drip rate.

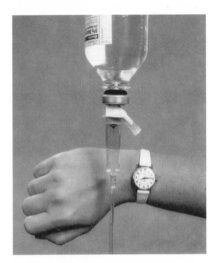

NURSING TIP If the clamp slips, for whatever reason, or the patient makes a sudden move, the drip rate may change. Check it periodically using the method described above. Remind the patient and his family not to tamper with the clamp.

Managing I.V. flow rate

Infusion pumps and controllers deliver precise amounts of fluids or medication to the patient by regulating the flow of I.V. solutions and agents. You'll use them when a precise flow rate is required, such as when administering total parenteral nutrition solutions and chemotherapeutic or cardiovascular agents. See Special Infusion Equipment for further discussion of pumps and controllers.

CORRECTING OBVIOUS FLOW RATE PROBLEMS

If an infusion is running too slowly or not at all, or an electronic infusion control device is beeping "occlusion" the problem may be easily corrected. Check to see if:

• the container's empty. Replace it.

• the drip chamber's less than half full. Squeeze it until the fluid reaches the proper level.

• the flow clamp's closed. Readjust it to restore the proper drip rate.

• the tubing's kinked or caught under the patient. Untangle the line or reposition the patient.

• the container is less than 3' (90 cm) above the site. Adjust the I.V. pole.

• the tubing is dangling below the site and gravity is preventing the flow of solution. Replace the tubing with a shorter piece, or tape some of the excess tubing to the I.V. pole (just below the flow clamp). Don't kink the tubing accidentally.

• an air bubble is in the tubing. Tap the tubing until the bubble rises into the container.

Understanding volume-control sets and filters

An alternative to mini bags, a volume-control set is an I.V. line featuring a fluid chamber that allows you to accurately deliver medication diluted in precise amounts of fluid. It's particularly useful for administering medications to children, particularly neonates, when the smallest inaccuracy can be lethal.

If your neonatal patient needs I.V. therapy, you'll probably use a vol-ume-control set as the *primary* I.V. line. You'll seldom use the set for a primary I.V. line in an adult; instead you'll connect it to a secondary port of an existing line. Use the volume-control set only when it's absolutely necessary, because it's costly and easily contaminated.

Before you establish an I.V. line with a volume-control set, make sure you know which filter the set features. You'll find either a membrane filter or a floating valve filter.

Both filters work effectively, but differ in structure. The membrane filter is rigid and remains stationary at the bottom of the fluid chamber. The floating valve filter is hinged on one side. This hinge allows it to move up and down with changes in fluid chamber pressure.

FLOW REGULATORS

By delivering a specific number of milliliters per hour, flow regulators help ensure accurate delivery of I.V. fluids. Less accurate than pumps or controllers, flow regulators are most reliable with inactive patients.

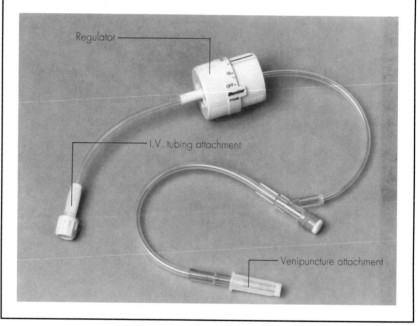

Regulator

I.V. tubing attachment

Venipuncture attachment

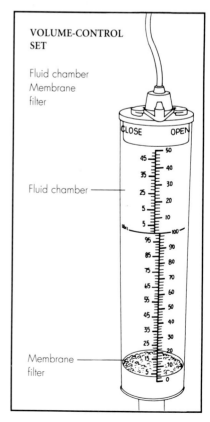

VOLUME-CONTROL SET

Fluid chamber
Membrane filter

Fluid chamber

Membrane filter

How to use a volume-control set with a membrane filter

1 Open the fluid chamber air vent. Then close the upper slide clamp, as shown.

Now, push the lower clamp to a point just below the drip chamber and close it. Remember, don't leave both main clamps open. Otherwise you'll get an unregulated fluid flow.

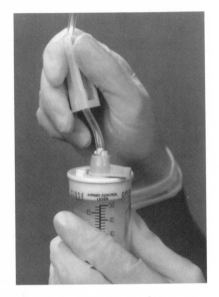

2 Wipe the top of the solution container with alcohol.

Remove the guard from the spike on the volume-control set, and insert the spike into the container. Then, hang the set.

3 Open the set's upper clamp, and squeeze the fluid chamber until it's filled with approximately 30 ml of solution. Close the upper clamp.

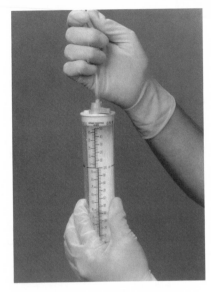

4 Squeeze the drip chamber until it's half full.

NURSING TIP If the drip chamber overfills, immediately close the upper clamp and the air vent. Then, invert the fluid chamber, and squeeze the excess solution from the drip chamber back into the fluid chamber. Don't wet the air vent filter or it may not work properly.

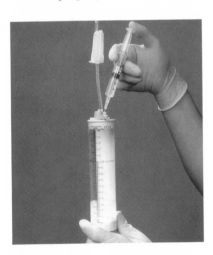

5 Remove the cover from the needle adapter, open the line's lower clamp, and prime the tubing and needle. Then, close the clamp again. Reattach the cover and the needle adapter.

Now you're ready to add medication to the line. Wipe the medication port on the fluid chamber with alcohol.

6 Draw the medication into a syringe. Then inject it into the fluid chamber making sure there's at least 30 ml of solution in the chamber. That will make mixing easier.

Now, label the fluid chamber with the dose of medication, but don't write directly on the plastic with a felt-tip marker. The ink could be absorbed through the plastic chamber and contaminate the medication. Instead, write on a narrow label or tape strip.

As needed, open the line's upper clamp, and fill the fluid chamber with the prescribed amount of solution. Then, close the upper clamp again, and gently rotate the fluid chamber until the solution is well mixed.

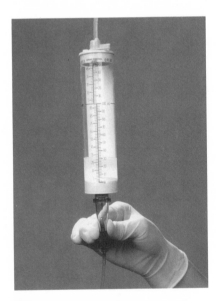

7 Wipe the injection port on the primary tubing with alcohol. This step's important because the port's exposed to contaminants.

COMPARING I.V. ADMINISTRATION SETS

I.V. administration sets are available in three major types: basic, add-a-line, and volume control. The basic set is used to administer most I.V. solutions. An add-a-line set delivers an intermittent secondary infusion through one or more injection sites. A volume-control set delivers small, precise amounts of solution. All three types are available with vented or nonvented drip chambers, depending on the type of solution container being used. (Glass containers require a vented drip chamber; plastic containers don't.)

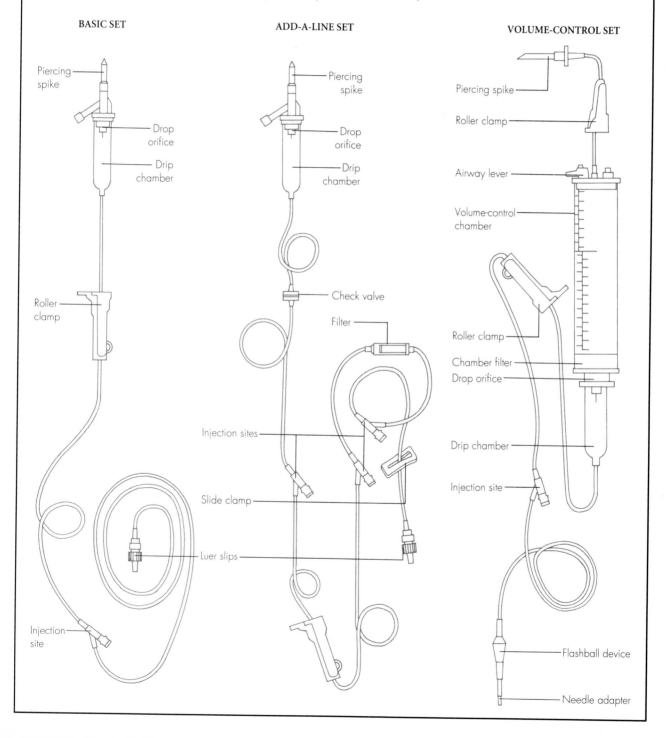

BASIC SET

Piercing spike

Drop orifice

Drip chamber

Roller clamp

Luer slips

Injection site

ADD-A-LINE SET

Piercing spike

Drop orifice

Drip chamber

Check valve

Filter

Injection sites

Slide clamp

VOLUME-CONTROL SET

Piercing spike

Roller clamp

Airway lever

Volume-control chamber

Roller clamp

Chamber filter

Drop orifice

Drip chamber

Injection site

Flashball device

Needle adapter

AVOIDING COMMON I.V. PROBLEMS

The best way to avoid I.V. complications is to learn the proper procedures *before* starting therapy. Otherwise, you could face various problems. The four most common are detailed below.

COMPLICATION	POSSIBLE CAUSES	SIGNS AND SYMPTOMS	NURSING CONSIDERATIONS
Infiltration	• Needle displacement (either partial or complete) • Leakage of blood around needle (especially in an older patient whose tissues have lost elasticity)	• Coolness of skin around site • Swelling around site • If a tourniquet's applied above the site, the infusion continues to run • Sluggish flow rate • Blood backflow may or may not be present	• Discontinue the infusion, and remove the needle immediately. • If the swelling's small, apply ice. Otherwise, apply warm wet compresses. • Restart I.V. in another limb. • Document your actions.
Thrombophlebitis	• Injury to the vein, either during venipuncture or subsequent needle movement • Irritation to the vein caused by long-term therapy, irritating or incompatible additives, or use of a vein that's too small for the amount or type of solution • Sluggish flow rate, which allows a clot to form at the end of the needle or catheter	• Tenderness and some redness at tip of venipuncture device, progressing to a vein that's sore, cordlike, and warm to the touch (may look like a red line above the venipuncture site) • Edematous site	• Discontinue the infusion, and remove the needle immediately. • Apply warm wet compresses. • Notify doctor. • Restart I.V. in another limb. • Document your actions. • *Important:* Never try to irrigate the line. In addition to increasing the risk of infection, you may flush a clot into the bloodstream, creating an embolus.
Systemic infection	• Poor aseptic technique • Contamination of equipment during manufacture, storage, or use • Traumatic venipuncture • Irrigation of clogged I.V.	• Sudden rise in temperature and pulse rate • Chills and shaking • Blood pressure changes	• Discontinue the I.V. immediately. Send equipment to the laboratory for bacterial analysis. • Look for other sources of infection. Culture urine, sputum, and blood, as ordered. • Restart I.V. in another limb. • Document your actions.
Speed shock	• Drugs administered too quickly • Improper administration of bolus infusions	• Headache • Tightness in chest • Irregular pulse rate • Shock, cardiac arrest	• Discontinue drug infusion. • Begin infusing dextrose 5% in water at a keep-vein-open rate. • Notify doctor immediately. • Document your actions.

HOW TO REPLACE I.V. EQUIPMENT   **99**

Insert the volume-control set needle. Use a 1" (5.1 cm) needle so you don't puncture the primary line. Secure the connection with tape as shown.

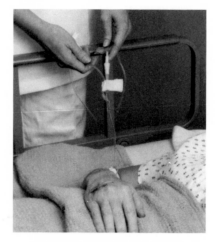

Turn off the primary I.V. line, or set it at a keep-vein-open rate. Then, open the lower clamp on the volume-control set, adjust the rate, and let the medication flow. Document the procedure and your observations.

Pediatric I.V. therapy

Because a child's anatomy and physiology differ significantly from an adult's, the child who must receive I.V. therapy needs special care. First of all, smaller size makes his system less tolerant of fluid and medication overdoses. Second, a child's metabolic rate is about three times faster than an adult's. Because that rate determines the body's water requirements, a child needs much more water.

The doctor considers these factors, along with weight, size, and clinical condition, when he calculates the amount to be administered intravenously. You can help by taking baseline readings, keeping accurate intake and output records, and watching for complications. Keep in mind that changes occur rapidly in

children. Up-to-date pediatric records are essential.

You'll administer pediatric I.V. therapy with an electronically controlled device or with a volume-control set. Because medication doses for children are more precise, make every effort to deliver all the medication in the fluid chamber.

Remember, I.V. therapy will probably be a new and frightening experience for the child, so give him all the attention and support you can. Explain the procedure in words he can understand. Answer his questions honestly. When the procedure's over, remember to compliment the child on his good behavior.

What about the parents?

An important part of your care of a child who's receiving I.V. therapy is the way you deal with the child's parents. The younger the child, the more he depends on his parents for support and the more their moods will influence how he feels. For example, if his parents are confused and uneasy, the child may be too. So be sure to include the parents in your patient teaching sessions. Once you reassure them and they understand the procedure, they can comfort and support their child more effectively.

If the parents want to, let them assist you in caring for the child. Encourage them to stay with the child during and after I.V. therapy procedures. But don't ask them to restrain the child or help you in any way during venipuncture.

How to replace I.V. equipment

The Centers for Disease Control in Atlanta recommends changing peripheral needles, catheters, and tubing every 72 hours, bags and bottles every 24 hours. Whenever possible, change the tubing and the container together. Remember, the more you handle the equipment, the greater the chance of contamination.

Occasionally, you'll have to be flexible. For example, if your patient has few available veins, you may have to leave a catheter in place longer than 72 hours. If so, be especially alert for signs of infection and infiltration.

On the following pages, you'll learn how to change the tubing and container together. As always, begin with a thorough hand washing.

1   Assemble a complete set of equipment, including tubing, container, dressings, and tape. Spike the container, prime the tubing, close the flow clamp, and cap the line (see How to Spike and Prime I.V. Solutions, pages 79 to 81).

To minimize your exposure to blood and other body fluids, always wear gloves when changing the I.V. tubing.

2   Remove the tape. To avoid dislodging the needle or catheter as you work, hold the needle hub with one hand while you remove the tape with the other hand as shown. Then, ask the patient not to move unnecessarily until everything is retaped.

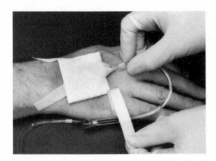

3   If the site dressing is soiled, wet, or loose, remove the dressing. Clean the skin around the venipuncture site with an antiseptic such as povidone-iodine solution (Betadine) or an alcohol pad. Then stabilize the

catheter. Place a fresh adhesive bandage or a transparent semipermeable dressing over the site.

4   To change the I.V. tubing, close the flow clamp on the old tubing, and place a 4" × 4" sterile gauze pad under the hub to create a sterile field. Then, press one of your fingers over the catheter to prevent bleeding, as shown. Grasp the hub with the sterile gauze pad to prevent touch contamination, and carefully disconnect the old adapter. If you hold the end of the new tubing between your fingers, as shown, you can insert it quickly.

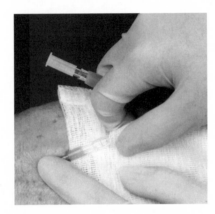

5   Remove the protective cap from the new tubing adapter. Working quickly, connect the adapter to the needle hub, as shown.

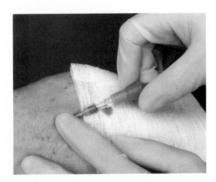

6   Secure the catheter, using the chevron taping method described on pages 89 and 90. Label the dressing with the type of needle in place, the

date of insertion, the date of dressing change, and your initials. Then readjust the flow rate.

NURSING TIP   Write the necessary information on the tape *before* you place it on the dressing, not after it's on the patient.

7   Label the container, as instructed on page 81, and document the entire procedure.

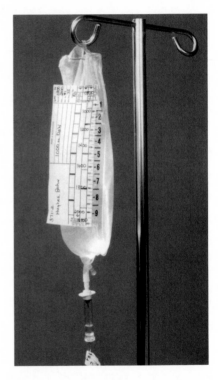

Replacing I.V. tubing

Sometimes you need to replace I.V. tubing without changing the existing bag or bottle. Before you begin, check the dressing and the site. Change the dressing according to your institution's policy.

1   Slow the infusion to the minimal flow rate, or keep-vein-open rate. Next, disconnect the old tubing from the bag and either hang it on the I.V. pole hook, as shown, or tape it to the pole. Loosely cover the end of the disconnected tubing with the spike cover from the new tubing. Remember, the other end is still connected to the patient, so take care to maintain sterile technique.

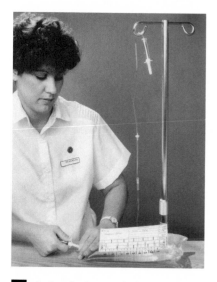

2 Spike the bag with the new tubing. Quickly flush the tubing and close the clamp. Then, carefully disconnect the old tubing from the insertion site connector.

3 Remove the protective cap from the new tubing and quickly insert the tubing adapter into the needle or catheter hub. Readjust the flow rate. Label the tubing and document the entire procedure.

I.V. Drug Administration

How to administer intermittent I.V. therapy using a heparin lock

The patient who doesn't require continuous I.V. infusion may require I.V. solutions and medications administered intermittently. To accommodate this, the doctor may order an existing I.V. line converted to a heparin lock.

1 Confirm the patient's identity by checking the name, room number, and bed number on his wristband. Then explain the procedure and why intermittent I.V. therapy is needed. This will help ease anxiety and encourage cooperation. Explain that intermittent I.V. therapy is administered by inserting a special device with an adapter plug. (If an I.V. line is not in place, see Performing Venipuncture.) Remember to wash your hands before beginning this procedure and to wear gloves when in direct patient contact.

As shown, male adapter plugs may be short or long with a luer or slip design. Such venipuncture devices may be referred to as heparin locks, prn adapters, intermittents, or INT'S.

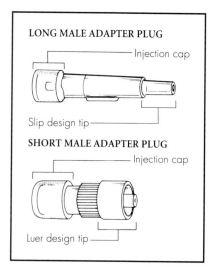

LONG MALE ADAPTER PLUG
— Injection cap
Slip design tip —

SHORT MALE ADAPTER PLUG
— Injection cap
Luer design tip —

2 The male adapter plug allows easy conversion of an I.V. line into a heparin lock for intermittent infusion of a medication. To convert, prime the male adapter plug with dilute heparin. Then clamp the I.V. tubing, remove the I.V. administration set from the catheter or needle hub, and insert the male adapter plug, as shown on the hand. Next, inject the remaining dilute heparin to fill the line and prevent clot formation.

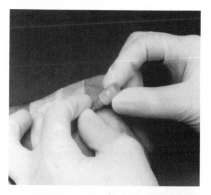

Refer to your institution's policy on maintaining heparin lock patency because these procedures vary among institutions.

3 To administer the prescribed medication or solution, attach a 20G 1" (2.5 cm) needle, a recessed needle, or a needleless system to the end of the I.V. tubing (any regular I.V. tubing can be used). Next, carefully clean the injection cap system with an alcohol pad. Then insert the needle into the injection cap as shown on page 102. Be sure to secure the needle or needleless system with tape to prevent dislodgment of the heparin lock. Now, adjust the flow rate to administer the medication over the specified infusion time. Remember to carefully inspect the venipuncture site for evidence of infiltration.

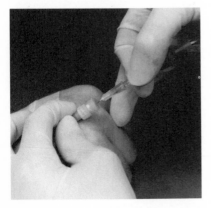

4 When the infusion is completed, remove the needle or needleless system from the heparin lock. Remove the needle or needleless system from the I.V. tubing and discard it appropriately. Then attach a new sterile needle with cap or a new needleless system to the end of the I.V. tubing. Now, flush the injection cap according to your institution's policy. You may use saline, dilute heparin, or both to flush the system. The flushing procedure will keep the I.V. catheter patent and will prepare the heparin lock for reuse. Document your actions in your nurse's notes.

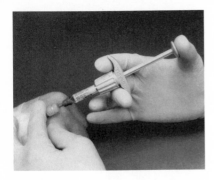

For this photo, a prefilled unit dose system was used to flush the injection cap.

GUIDELINES FOR HEPARINIZATION OF INTERMITTENT INFUSION

Because fluid does not flow continuously through an intermittent infusion device, a special procedure called heparinization must be performed after each use to ensure patency. The following heparinization procedure, known as SASH, is used at some institutions:

• **S** = saline 2 ml. Inject normal saline solution into the cannula to flush the previously injected solution and prevent the mixing of medications.

• **A** = antibiotic or admixture. Perform the required procedure, such as infusing piggyback medication or withdrawing blood. If blood is drawn, the first 3 to 5 ml will be diluted. Discard and take another sample.

• **S** = saline 2 ml. Flush cannula again with this solution.

• **H** = heparin flush. Inject 1 ml diluted heparin solution (usually 100 U/ml or 10 U/ml) into the cannula to prevent thrombus formation in the cannula and at its tip.

Investigators are trying to determine if flushing with normal saline solution alone is sufficient to maintain patency in heparin locks. This would eliminate the need for routine heparinization. Depending on the results of these studies, flushing with saline alone may become routine.

Flushing heparin locks

When you inject medication into a heparin lock, a small amount will remain in the cannula. Flushing the cannula with normal saline solution will ensure that the patient receives the entire dose.

When discontinuing the lock after injecting medication, flush the cannula with normal saline solution before removing it. This will remove all vesicants or irritating solutions from the cannula tip. Even the smallest amount of some medications can severely irritate or damage tissue.

Although only 1 to 2 ml of solution may remain in the cannula after an injection, precipitation can still result if the solution is not compatible with the next medication. A saline flush will prevent medication from mixing in the cannula.

HEPARIN PRACTICE SURVEY

Recommended practices for maintaining patency of a heparin lock vary depending on the institution in which you work. According to results of a nationwide practice survey, 40% of the respondents use 100 U/ml of heparin to flush heparin locks, 37% use 10 U/ml of heparin, and 18% use normal saline. The remaining 5% use other solutions or dilutions.

The survey also showed 96% of respondents use heparinized flush solutions for arterial lines in the critical care setting. Almost 90% use heparinized saline, 6% use heparinized glucose, and 1% use heparinized lactate solutions. Only 2% use plain saline or glucose.

How are heparinization policies set? About half of the respondents base their policy on custom, 17% on doctor, manufacturer, or pharmacy recommendations, and 20% were unsure of the policy's origin.

How to use a T-connector

To administer fluids and drugs simultaneously or to administer a medication that is incompatible with the primary I.V. solution, you may want to use a special piece of I.V. equipment called a T-connector, shown below. This small-bore extension tubing is 3" to 6" (7.6 to 15.2 cm) long and has an injection site near its luer connection. This added injection site can also serve as an intermittent infusion device (heparin lock) while the primary I.V. solution infuses. The device often eliminates the need for insertion of a second venipuncture device. The slide clamp on the extension set allows the primary solution to be shut off during infusion of an incompatible solution.

Adding the T-connector

1 Wash your hands and put on gloves to minimize exposure to body fluids. Then, explain to the patient what you are about to do. An additional piece of I.V. equipment may cause your patient to be alarmed, so explaining this procedure before you begin should ease the patient's anxiety. Now, attach the one end of the T-connector to the I.V. tubing as shown and open the slide clamp.

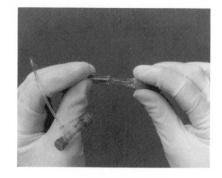

Next, prime the tubing with I.V. fluid.

2 Now you are ready to connect the luer tip to the existing I.V. cannula. (To insert an I.V. cannula and prime an I.V. line, refer to How to Spike and Prime I.V. Solutions, pages 79 to 81. Remove the luer tip protector cap and carefully insert this tip into the I.V. cannula as shown.

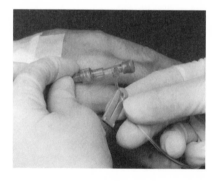

Secure this connector in place with tape. Another I.V. needle can be inserted into the latex injection cap. Finally, document your actions.

How to mix secondary I.V. infusions

If your institution's pharmacy does not prepare I.V. infusions for secondary administration, you can use the following procedure.

1 Read the medication package insert. If you need to reconstitute the medication, follow the steps on pages 62 and 63. Then, draw up the medication with a filter needle and syringe. Remember, you can use a filter needle only once. Replace it with a large-bore (18G) 1½" (3.8 cm) needle before injecting medication into the secondary container.

2 Swab the bag's secondary medication port with alcohol. Then, inject the medication into the port. Gently rotate it to mix the solution.

3 Affix a *medication-added* label to the container. Include the drug dose, date and time, expiration date (if pertinent), patient's name, and room and bed number. Remember to initial it.

4 Attach the tubing to the secondary bag by driving the spike into the bag. Hang the set.

NOTE Some medications now come in vials suitable for hanging directly on an I.V. pole. Instead of preparing medication and injecting it into a container, you can inject diluent directly into the medication vial. Then, spike the vial, prime the tubing, and hang the set as usual.

5 Attach a 20G 1" (2.5 cm) needle to the tubing adapter and prime the entire secondary set.

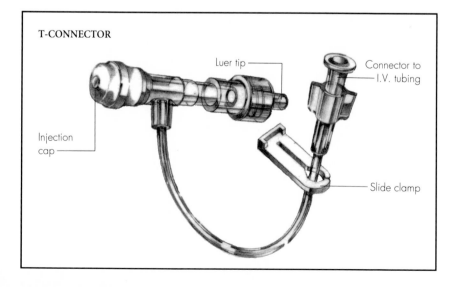

T-CONNECTOR

Luer tip

Connector to I.V. tubing

Injection cap

Slide clamp

HANGING ADDITIVE SETS

Sometimes you must administer I.V. medication to a patient with a primary I.V. line in place. If the drug can't be mixed with the primary solution or you must give it slowly or intermittently, you'll use an additive set.

A *piggyback set* includes a small I.V. bag or bottle, short tubing, and usually a macrodrip system. This set connects into a primary line's upper Y port, also called the piggyback port. A piggyback set is used solely for intermittent drug administration. To make this set work, you must position the primary I.V. container below the piggyback container (the manufacturer provides an extension hook for that purpose).

A *secondary set* features an I.V. bag or bottle (any size), long tubing, and either a microdrip or a macrodrip system. The set connects into the primary line's lower Y port, which is also called the secondary port. A secondary set is used to administer drugs intermittently or simultaneously with a primary solution.

PRIMARY AND PIGGYBACK SETS   **PRIMARY AND SECONDARY SETS**

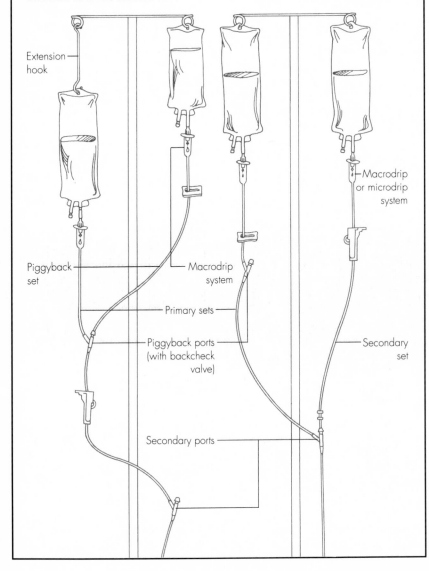

Extension hook

Piggyback set

Macrodrip system

Primary sets

Piggyback ports (with backcheck valve)

Secondary ports

Macrodrip or microdrip system

Secondary set

When administering two drugs simultaneously, be sure to consult a compatibility chart or your institution's pharmacist to check if these drugs may infuse concurrently into a single I.V. site.

Make sure the medication's compatible with the primary line solution. If it *isn't*, swab the secondary port with alcohol. Then, flush the primary tubing with saline solution before inserting the set's needle.

If the medication *is* compatible, simply swab the secondary port with alcohol and insert the 20G 1" needle. Secure this device into the port with tape.

Begin infusing the medication at the prescribed rate. Follow the doctor's orders; he may want it to run separately or with the primary solution. Document what you've done.

ADDITIVE SETS: INDICATIONS AND CONTRAINDICATIONS

When a patient with a primary I.V. line also requires intermittent medication administration, use an I.V. additive set.

It will enable you to:
• Maintain peak drug levels in the patient's bloodstream
• Avoid irritation from I.V. bolus
• Administer different drugs at different times.

Two of the most common drugs administered in this way are antibiotics and H_2 antagonists.

However, never use an I.V. additive set when the drug you're giving must be given slowly or well-diluted, such as vitamins or KCl.

ADDITIVE SETS: ALTERNATIVE EQUIPMENT

The following photos show alternative equipment you might use when preparing additive sets. To review the procedures for using volume-control sets, see How to Use a Volume-Control Set with a Membrane Filter, pages 96 to 99.

The partial-fill piggyback set procedure requires a minibag or minibottle, macro-drip tubing, an 18G or 19G 1" (2.5 cm) needle, an extension hook, and a medication-added label.

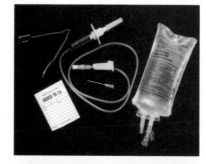

The ADD-Vantage System requires an 18G or 19G 1" needle, volume-control tubing, and dextrose 5% in water (D_5W).

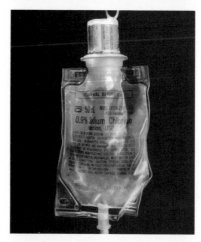

The volume-control set procedure requires an 18G or 19G 1" needle, volume-control tubing, and D_5W.

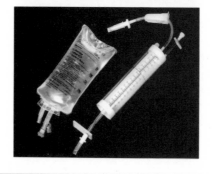

CARING FOR A PATIENT WITH AN ADDITIVE SET

Before using an additive set, explain to the patient why you're hanging another bottle. Tell him how it works, and answer his questions honestly to help minimize fears and make him more comfortable.

Stay alert for signs of drug sensitivity, especially after the first dose. To read his reaction accurately, you'll need to establish reference points by getting the answers to these questions before you start:
• What are the patient's known allergies?
• Does he have a skin condition (such as hives) that makes drug sensitivity difficult to assess?
• Is he uncomfortable or experiencing chills?
• What's his urine output?
• What's his temperature, pulse rate, respiratory rate, and blood pressure?

If his condition seems to contraindicate the drug, check with the doctor before you administer it.

During administration, watch the patient closely for signs of drug sensitivity. If he shows any, discontinue the drug immediately and call a doctor. When you complete administration, assess the patient's condition again. Because you've established reference points, you can accurately judge the drug's effects.

How to use a partial-fill piggyback set

If your patient needs intermittent infusion of a diluted drug, you can use a partial-fill piggyback set to deliver it. If your institution's pharmacy doesn't prepare partial-fill piggyback sets, follow these steps:

1 Begin the partial-fill piggyback procedure by following the steps for adding medication to a primary I.V. line. Swab the medication port with alcohol. Read the directions. If the drug should be reconstituted, see pages 62 and 63. If it's ready for use, draw the solution into a syringe. Then, insert the needle into the partial-fill piggyback container and inject the medication.

2   Label the piggyback bag with the following information: the medication added, the date and time of addition, and your initials. Be sure you invert the label so it's right side up when the bag's hung, as shown. If the pharmacy mixed the solution, the container will be labeled with the appropriate information. Make sure this matches the information on the medication order.

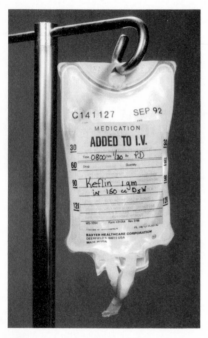

3   Close the piggyback line flow clamp. Insert the spike into the container (see pages 79 and 80).

4   If you are using a needle, a needle attachment may be included in the piggyback set. If it's not, attach an 18G or 19G 1" (2.5 cm) needle to the line. Don't use a needle longer than 1" because it will puncture the tubing. Connect the needle to the secondary tubing. Open the flow clamp for a few seconds to prime the tubing and needle attachment. Then close it again. Now insert the needle of the

USING A NEEDLE LOCK DEVICE FOR SECONDARY LINES

In this device, the needle is recessed to prevent accidental needle sticks and surrounded by a protective locking shield. It's available alone, or as part of a secondary medication set and fits any luer-lock adapter. Once the secondary set is attached, twist the lock a half-turn, as shown in the inset, to prevent dislodgment.

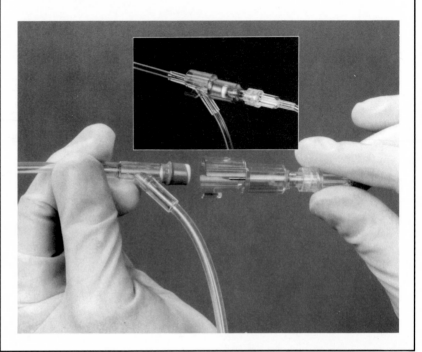

piggyback tubing into the continuous flow secondary port.

5   Label the secondary tubing with the date and time you established the line as shown. *Remember:* Replace piggyback tubing according to your institution's policy. The Centers for Disease Control recommends changing piggyback tubing every 72 hours.

Make sure the medication you're administering is compatible with the primary I.V. solution. If it's not, you must flush the primary I.V. line with saline solution before connecting the piggyback set needle to the port. Tape it securely or use a needle lock device.

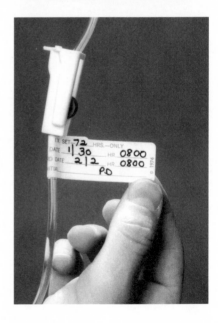

6 Now you're ready to infuse the partial-fill piggyback with a continuous flow set. With this system, the piggyback will infuse while the primary I.V. is temporarily stopped.

Use the extension hook to rehang the primary container. Its center of gravity must be lower than the minibag's, as shown.

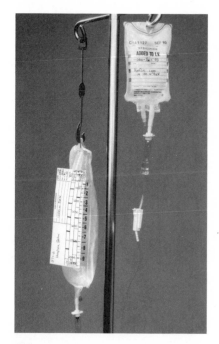

7 Open the piggyback line flow clamp. Because the minibag is placed higher than the primary container, the backcheck valve will automatically cut off the flow of *primary* solution and allow the medication to flow. Adjust the flow to the medication's recommended rate.

8 When the piggyback solution level drops below the drip chamber of the primary container, the backcheck valve cuts off the *piggyback* flow. Then, the primary solution automatically begins running again.

NOTE To administer the piggyback solution that remains in the piggyback tubing, pinch the primary tubing closed just above the piggy-

back port. This allows the piggyback solution to drain. Watch it carefully.

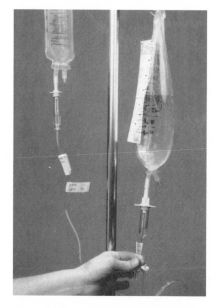

At the moment the tubing empties, release your pressure on the tubing. This will allow the primary solution to run again, perhaps even filling part of the piggyback line. However, the backcheck valve will prevent the primary solution from entering the piggyback bag.

> **When the primary solution is running again, readjust its flow to the prescribed rate; otherwise, it will flow at the piggyback rate.**

9 When you're ready to hang a *new* piggyback bag, follow these steps to clear the tubing of air. First, disconnect the old bag, and spike the new one. Then, open the clamp on the piggyback line, and lower the bag below the backcheck valve. This will cause primary fluid to run up the piggyback tubing and will expel any trapped air into the bottle. Finally, hang the piggyback bag above the

primary container, and adjust the flow rate.

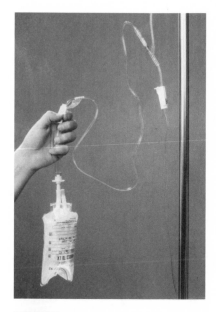

NOTE Most piggyback solutions contain 50 to 100 ml of solution and medication. They are usually infused in 30 to 60 minutes. Some irritating medications require greater dilution and longer infusion times to minimize harmful local effects.

CRIS: Another way to deliver secondary I.V. drugs

IVAC's Controlled Release Infusion System (CRIS) offers an easy and cost-effective way to administer secondary drugs through a primary I.V. line. Connected to the I.V. line between the primary container and the administration set, the CRIS adapter lets you administer a drug dose without using a minibag and piggyback administration set. You simply attach a single-dose vial to the CRIS spike and turn the CRIS valve handle toward the vial. The primary infusion flows into the vial and mixes with the drug; the mixture then flows down the line to the patient. You can use the adapter with any I.V. solution container and any primary set.

Besides simplicity, CRIS offers these timesaving benefits:
• You needn't interrupt the primary flow to administer a secondary drug.
• You don't have to flush tubing between drugs.
• Because you use only one solution container, you can monitor fluid intake more easily.
• This system saves the time you'd ordinarily spend priming secondary sets, adjusting and readjusting primary and secondary flow rates, and handling secondary containers.
• This system saves the storage space you'd need for minibags and secondary I.V. sets.

Use the CRIS adapter with unvented I.V. tubing and reconstituted drugs in single-dose vials (from 5 to 20 ml).

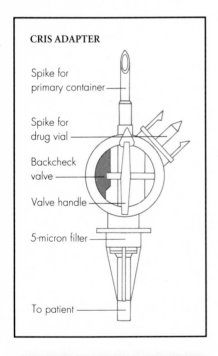

CRIS ADAPTER

Spike for primary container

Spike for drug vial

Backcheck valve

Valve handle

5-micron filter

To patient

For safe, effective use, read and follow the manufacturer's recommendations.

How to use a CRIS adapter

1 Install the CRIS adapter on the patient's I.V. line. *Push* the administration set's spike into the adapter's lower port, *don't twist*. Obtain a single-dose vial of reconstituted drug (as ordered) and an alcohol pad.

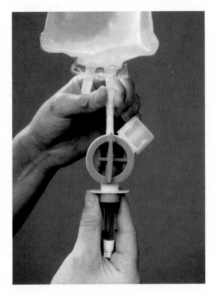

2 Remove the vial's temporary cover and clean its diaphragm with the alcohol pad. Using a twisting motion, remove the protective cover from the CRIS vial spike and impale the vial on the spike.

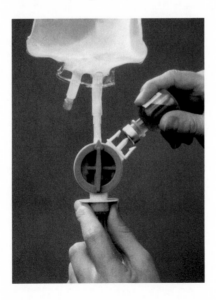

NURSING TIP If you encounter resistance, puncture the diaphragm with a needle to release air.

3 Make sure the primary container holds at least 60 ml of fluid (the volume needed to deliver the dose and flush the system). Then, to begin drug delivery, turn the valve handle toward the vial until you feel resistance. Click the valve into place in the 2 o'clock position.

Calculate the flow rate and set the pump appropriately, or mark or time tape the container.

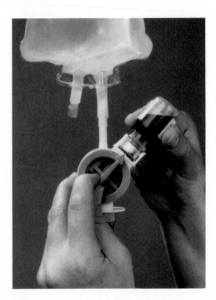

4 After drug delivery's complete, leave the vial in place and keep the valve handle in the 2 o'clock position until you're ready to deliver another drug dose. (Note that because the primary infusion flows through the vial, the vial doesn't empty.) Leaving the vial in place maintains the vial spike's sterility.

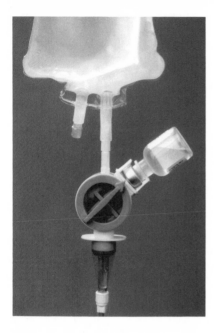

5 Before giving another drug dose, make sure the primary I.V. container holds at least 60 ml of fluid. Then turn the valve handle to the 12 o'clock position.

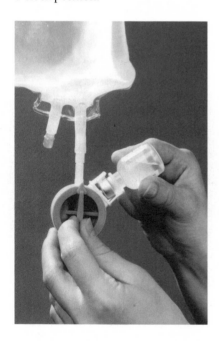

6 Adjust the drip chamber's fluid level, if necessary. If the vial is inadvertently pressurized during reconstitution, if the drug produces gas, or if the drip chamber is squeezed with the valve in the 2 o'clock position, the backcheck valve will prevent reflux of the drug solution into the primary conainer.

7 Remove the used vial and replace it with the new one, as described above.

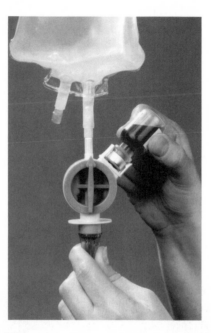

8 Turn the valve handle back to the 2 o'clock position. Adjust the flow rate, if necessary.

Change the CRIS adapter when you change the administration set, every 48 hours or according to institution policy.

NOTE You can use the CRIS adapter on a primary line while delivering another drug through a piggyback set.

How to cope with drug incompatibilities

If the drug you're administering is incompatible with the primary solution, follow these steps:

1 Mix the drug with a diluent, and draw it up into a syringe. Place the cap back on the needle and set the syringe aside. Then draw saline solution or dextrose 5% in water into two other syringes.

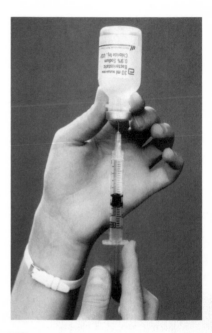

2 Close the roller clamp on the primary infusion set. Insert the needle of one of the saline-filled syringes into the line's secondary port. After checking for blood backflow, flush the tubing with saline solution.

Swab the port with alcohol and inject the medication. Don't open the roller clamp until you've flushed the tubing with the remaining saline-filled syringe.

(Text continues on page 114.)

RISKS OF PERIPHERAL I.V. THERAPY

Peripheral I.V. therapy carries associated risks of local and systemic complications. Remember that when you give a drug by the I.V. bolus method it will have an immediate effect. Pay special attention to the patient's reaction. If he's able to respond, ask him how he feels.

This chart lists some common complications with their signs and symptoms, possible causes, and nursing interventions, including prevention measures.

SIGNS AND SYMPTOMS	POSSIBLE CAUSES	NURSING INTERVENTIONS	PREVENTION MEASURES
Local Complications			
Phlebitis			
• Tenderness at tip of venipuncture device and above • Redness at tip of catheter and along vein • Puffy area over vein • Vein hard on palpation • Elevated temperature	• Poor blood flow around venipuncture device • Friction from catheter movement in vein • Venipuncture device left in vein too long • Clotting at catheter tip (thrombophlebitis) • Solution with high or low pH or high osmolarity	• Remove venipuncture device. • Apply warm pack. • Notify doctor if patient has fever. • Document patient's condition and your interventions.	• Restart infusion using larger vein for irritating infusate, or restart with smaller gauge device to ensure adequate blood flow. • Use filter to reduce risk of phlebitis. • Tape venipuncture device securely to prevent motion.
Extravasation			
• Swelling at and above I.V. site (may extend along entire limb) • Discomfort, burning, or pain at site • Feeling of tightness at site • Decreased skin temperature around site • Blanching at site • Continuing fluid infusion even when vein is occluded, although rate may decrease • Absent backflow of blood • Slower flow rate	• Venipuncture device dislodged from vein or perforated vein	• Remove venipuncture device. • Apply ice (early) or warm soaks (later) to aid absorption. • Elevate limb. • Check for pulse and capillary refill periodically to assess circulation. • Restart infusion above infiltration site or in another limb. • Document patient's condition and your interventions.	• Check I.V. site frequently (especially when using I.V. pump). • Don't obscure area above site with tape. • Teach patient to observe I.V. site and report pain or swelling.
Catheter dislodgment			
• Loose tape • Catheter partly backed out of vein • Infusate infiltrating	• Loosened tape or tubing snagged in bedclothes, resulting in partial retraction of catheter	• If no infiltration occurs, retape without pushing catheter back into vein.	• Tape venipuncture device securely on insertion.

RISKS OF PERIPHERAL I.V. THERAPY *continued*

SIGNS AND SYMPTOMS	POSSIBLE CAUSES	NURSING INTERVENTIONS	PREVENTION MEASURES
Local Complications continued			
Occlusion			
• No increase in flow rate when I.V. container is raised • Blood backup in line	• I.V. flow interrupted • Heparin lock not flushed • Blood backup in line when patient walks • Hypercoagulable patient • Line clamped too long	• Use mild flush injection. Don't force injection. If unsuccessful, reinsert I.V. line.	• Maintain I.V. flow rate. • Flush promptly after intermittent piggyback administration. • Have patient walk with his arm folded to chest to reduce risk of blood backup.
Vein irritation or pain			
• Pain during infusion • Possible blanching if vasospasm occurs • Red skin over vein during infusion • Rapidly developing signs of phlebitis	• Solution with high or low pH or high osmolarity, such as 40 mEq/liter of potassium chloride, phenytoin (Dilantin), and some antibiotics (vancomycin [Vancocin] and nafcillin [Nafcil])	• Slow the flow rate. • Try using an electronic flow device to achieve a steady flow.	• Dilute solutions before administration. For example, give antibiotics in 250 ml of solution rather than 100 ml. If drug has low pH, ask pharmacist if drug can be buffered with sodium bicarbonate (refer to policy). • If long-term therapy of irritating drug is planned, ask doctor to use central I.V. line.
Severed catheter			
• Leakage from catheter shaft	• Catheter inadvertently cut by scissors • Reinsertion of needle into catheter	• If broken part is visible, attempt to retrieve it. • If portion of catheter enters bloodstream, place tourniquet above I.V. site. • Notify doctor and radiology department. • Document patient's condition and your interventions.	• Don't use scissors around I.V. site. • Never reinsert needle into catheter. • Remove unsuccessfully inserted catheter and needle together.
Hematoma			
• Tenderness at venipuncture site • Area around site bruised • Inability to advance or flush I.V. line	• Vein punctured through other wall at time of venipuncture • Leakage of blood from needle displacement	• Remove venipuncture device. • Apply pressure and warm soaks to affected area. • Recheck for bleeding. • Document patient's condition and your interventions.	• Choose a vein that can accommodate size of venipunture device. • Release tourniquet as soon as successful insertion is achieved.

continued

RISKS OF PERIPHERAL I.V. THERAPY *continued*

SIGNS AND SYMPTOMS	POSSIBLE CAUSES	NURSING INTERVENTIONS	PREVENTION MEASURES
Local Complications continued			
Venous spasm			
• Pain along vein • Flow rate sluggish when clamp completely open • Blanched skin over vein	• Severe vein irritation from irritating drugs or fluids • Administration of cold fluids or blood • Very rapid flow rate (with fluid at room temperature)	• Apply warm soaks over vein and surrounding area. • Slow flow rate.	• Use blood warmer for blood or packed red blood cells.
Vasovagal reaction			
• Sudden collapse of vein during venipuncture • Sudden pallor accompanied by sweating, faintness, dizziness, and nausea • Decreased blood pressure	• Vasospasm from anxiety or pain	• Lower head of bed. • Have patient take deep breaths. • Check vital signs.	• Prepare patient adequately for therapy to relieve anxiety. • Use local anesthetic to prevent pain of venipuncture.
Thrombosis			
• Painful, reddened, and swollen vein • Sluggish or stopped I.V. flow	• Injury to endothelial cells of vein wall, allowing platelets to adhere and thrombus to form	• Remove venipuncture device; restart infusion in opposite limb if possible. • Apply warm soaks. • Watch for infection: thrombi provide an excellent environment for bacterial growth.	• Use proper venipuncture techniques to reduce injury to vein.
Thrombophlebitis			
• Severe discomfort • Reddened, swollen, and hardened vein	• Thrombosis and inflammation	• Same as for thrombosis.	• Check site frequently. Remove venipuncture device at first sign of redness and tenderness.

RISKS OF PERIPHERAL I.V. THERAPY *continued*

SIGNS AND SYMPTOMS	POSSIBLE CAUSES	NURSING INTERVENTIONS	PREVENTION MEASURES
Local Complications *continued*			
Nerve, tendon, or ligament damage			
• Extreme pain • Numbness and muscle contraction • Delayed effects (paralysis, numbness, and deformity)	• Improper venipuncture technique, resulting in injury to surrounding nerves, tendons, or ligaments • Tight taping or improper splinting with armboard	• Stop procedure.	• Avoid repeated venipuncture. • Don't apply excessive pressure when taping or encircle limb with tape. • Pad armboards and pad tape securing armboard if possible.
Systemic Complications			
Circulatory overload			
• Discomfort • Neck vein engorgement • Respiratory distress • Increased blood pressure • Crackles • Increased difference between fluid intake and output	• Roller clamp loosened to allow run-on infusion • Flow rate too rapid • Miscalculation of fluid requirements	• Raise the head of the bed. • Administer oxygen as needed. • Notify doctor. • Administer medications (such as diuretics) as ordered.	• Use pump, controller, or rate minder for elderly or compromised patients. • Recheck calculations of fluid requirements. • Monitor infusion frequently.
Systemic infection (septicemia or bacteremia)			
• Fever, chills, and malaise for no apparent reason • Contaminated I.V. site, usually with no visible signs of infection	• Failure to maintain aseptic technique • Severe phlebitis, creating conditions for organism growth • Poor taping that permits venipuncture device to move, introducing organisms into bloodstream • Prolonged use of venipuncture device • Immunocompromised patient	• Notify doctor. • Administer medications as prescribed. • Culture site and device. • Monitor vital signs.	• Use scrupulous aseptic technique when handling solutions and tubings, inserting venipuncture device, and discontinuing infusion. • Secure all connections. • Change I.V. solutions, tubing, and venipucture device at recommended times. • Use I.V. filters.
Speed shock			
• Flushed face • Headache • Tightness in chest • Irregular pulse • Syncope • Shock • Cardiac arrest	• Too rapid injection of drug, causing plasma concentration to reach toxic levels • Improper administration of bolus infusion (especially additives)	• Discontinue drug infusion. • Begin infusion of dextrose 5% in water at keep-vein-open rate. • Notify doctor immediately.	• Read medication insert on infusion recommendations before giving any medications.

continued

RISKS OF PERIPHERAL I.V. THERAPY *continued*

SIGNS AND SYMPTOMS	POSSIBLE CAUSES	NURSING INTERVENTIONS	PREVENTION MEASURES
Systemic Complications continued			
Air embolism			
• Respiratory distress • Unequal breath sounds • Weak pulse • Increased central venous pressure • Decreased blood pressure • Loss of consciousness	• Solution container empty • Solution container empties, and added container pushes air down line	• Discontinue infusion. • Place patient in Trendelenburg's position to allow air to enter right atrium and disperse via pulmonary artery. • Administer oxygen. • Notify doctor. • Document patient's condition and your interventions.	• Purge tubing of air completely before infusion. • Use air-detection device on pump or air-eliminating filter proximal to I.V. site. • Secure connections.
Allergic reaction			
• Itching • Tearing eyes and runny nose • Bronchospasm • Wheezing • Urticarial rash • Edema at I.V. site • Anaphylactic reaction (may occur within minutes or up to 1 hour after exposure), including flushing, chills, anxiety, agitation, generalized itching, palpitations, paresthesia, throbbing in ears, wheezing, coughing, seizures, and cardiac arrest	• Allergens such as medications	• If reaction occurs, stop infusion immediately. • Maintain patent airway. • Notify doctor. • Administer antihistaminic steroid, anti-inflammatory, and antipyretic drugs, as ordered. • Give 0.2 to 0.5 ml of 1:1,000 aqueous epinephrine subcutaneously. Repeat at 3-minute intervals and as needed. • Administer cortisone if ordered.	• Obtain patient's allergy history. Be aware of cross-allergies. • Assist with test dosing. • Monitor patient carefully during first 15 minutes of administration of a new drug.

3 An alternative to giving incompatible drugs with the primary solution is the addition of a T-connector to the distal end of the tubing as shown here. A T-connector allows simultaneous or intermittent administration. Simply flush the T-connector and administer the drug via the injection port on the T-connector while the primary infusion continues.

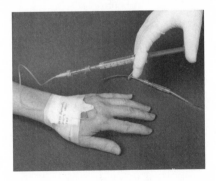

NOTE Drugs may be compatible if not mixed in the same solution or if, once mixed, they're infused within a specified time. If in doubt, ask the pharmacist if drugs can be safely piggybacked in the tubing of a continuously infusing I.V. or with a T-connector. If no compatibility data exists, always administer the drugs separately.

Central Venous Infusion

Selecting a central venous infusion device

First used only 40 years ago, central venous infusion devices are now in common use. An estimated 3 million such devices are used annually in the United States alone.

Selecting the most appropriate device for a particular patient requires a collaborative decision involving the patient, the doctor, and the nurse. This decision should take into account the indication, the types of catheters available for that purpose, as well as each catheter's properties and potential complications. It should also take into account the patient's ability to manage catheter self-care, and the patient's projected needs for other therapies.

Forms of central venous catheters

Central venous catheters are available in three basic forms: the over-the-needle catheter (ONC), the through the needle catheter, and the most commonly used form, the catheter threaded over a guidewire. The catheter's basic form, what it's made of, and its intended uses determine which is most appropriate for a given patient. Central venous catheters are made of polyurethane, polyvinyl chloride, or silicone rubber for either short- or long-term use.

Short-term catheters

Catheters designed for short-term use include single or multiple lumen catheters of polyurethane or polyvinyl chloride. The multiple lumen catheters allow simultaneous administration of more than one solution without regard for compatibility. Lumen sizes vary depending on the manufacturer. Commonly, the multiple lumen catheter has three lumens, one 16G distal lumen and two 18G proximal and medial lumens. The lumens open into the central vein at approximately 5" (12.7 cm) intervals. These catheters are slightly stiff, allowing speedier insertion over a guidewire. Many multiple lumen catheters have a heparin coating to prevent clot formation. Check the package insert for information on the catheter you are using.

These catheters usually are not recommended for prolonged therapy because the stiffness of the catheter may irritate the vessel and increase the risk of infection from catheter movement at the insertion site. Because of these risks, the Intravenous Nurses Society recommends that these catheters be changed every 3 to 7 days.

Long-term catheters

Catheters designed for long-term use are more flexible and are usually made of silicone rubber (Silastic), which is less thrombogenic because it is more compatible physiologically. Examples of silicone rubber long-term central venous catheters include the Hickman, Broviac, and Groshong catheters.

Because these catheters are also more flexible, insertion may be more difficult and is usually performed in the operating room. With a cutdown procedure, the catheter is inserted directly into a central vein. When the catheter tip is in the vein, the remaining catheter is placed into the subcutaneous tissue and threaded (tunneled) to an exit site on the skin surface. The catheter may be cut to size during the procedure to prevent

---

CENTRAL VENOUS INFUSION: PROS AND CONS

Central venous infusion is the administration of fluid through an I.V. catheter placed in a central vein. With cannulation of the subclavian vein and internal and external jugular veins, the catheter tip rests in the superior vena cava. With the femoral vein, the catheter tip rests in the inferior vena cava.

In peripheral central venous therapy, the central catheter is inserted in a peripheral vein, usually the basilic or cephalic vein. The catheter's distal tip terminates in the superior vena cava.

Pros
- Eliminates need for multiple peripheral venipuncture.
- Provides access to central venous circulation for rapid infusion of large amounts of fluid.
- Decreases risk of vein irritation from infusion of caustic substances.
- Provides a means for measuring central venous pressure as an indicator of circulatory function.
- Allows preservation or restoration of peripheral veins.

Cons
- Increases risk of complications, such as sepsis, thrombus formation, and perforation of an adjacent organ.
- Decreases patient's mobility when certain sites are used.
- Insertion requires more time and higher level of skill.
- Increases cost of equipment.

CENTRAL VENOUS INFUSION SITES

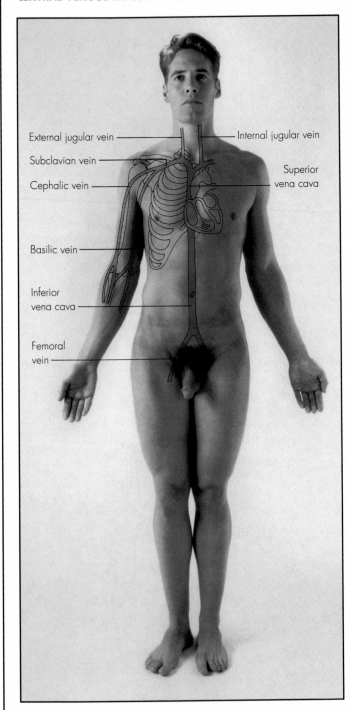

External jugular vein
Subclavian vein
Cephalic vein
Internal jugular vein
Superior vena cava
Basilic vein
Inferior vena cava
Femoral vein

SITE	ADVANTAGES
Internal jugular vein	• Short, direct route to right atrium • Catheter stability • Less movement with respirations • Less risk of pneumothorax
External jugular vein	• Easy access, especially in children • Less risk of pneumothorax or arterial puncture
Subclavian vein	• Easy access • Easy to keep dressing in place • High blood flow rates make thrombus formation unlikely
Cephalic vein	• Relatively easy access • Minimal risk of major complications • Easy to keep dressing in place
Basilic vein	• Easy access • Direct, straight course to superior vena cava • Minimal risk of major complications • Easy to keep dressing in place
Femoral vein	• Good site for children and elderly patients • Relatively easy access

DISADVANTAGES

- Close proximity to common carotid
- Position on neck makes sterile dressing difficult to maintain
- Potential for tracheal lacerations and punctures

- Less direct route
- Lower blood flow rates may increase risk of thrombus formation
- Difficult to keep dressing in place
- Vein may be tortuous, especially in elderly patients

- Potential for pneumothorax
- Possible laceration of subclavian artery
- Difficult to control bleeding (noncompressable vessel)

- Antecubital fossa difficult to locate in obese patients
- Difficult to keep elbow immobile, especially in children
- Not a straight course to superior vena cava

- Antecubital fossa difficult to locate in obese patients
- Difficult to keep elbow immobile, especially in children
- Close proximity to brachial artery

- Difficult to keep dressing intact
- Decreased patient mobility
- Increased potential for thrombus formation
- Difficult to cannulate in obese patients

excess length on the outside. Just before the point where the catheter exits the skin, the doctor positions a polyester fabric (Dacron) cuff. Granulation tissue forms around this cuff in about 2 weeks, helping to secure the catheter and acting as a barrier to organism migration.

Also considered a long-term catheter, the peripherally inserted central catheter (PICC) is placed percutaneously through the cephalic or basilic veins in the arm. It is then threaded into the superior vena cava (see Learning about the Peripherally Inserted Central Catheter, page 130).

Another type of long-term central venous catheter uses an implanted port for infusions (see Learning about Subcutaneous Access Devices, page 153).

For additional information about long-term central venous catheters, see *Comparing central venous infusion devices,* pages 118 to 121.

Preparing the patient for insertion of a central venous catheter

Ensuring the patient's cooperation and compliance with insertion of a central venous catheter requires your ability to enhance the doctor's explanation of the procedure and its related complications in terms the patient can understand. You must know enough about the procedure to answer the patient's questions regarding the purpose and expected outcome of the procedure as well as the patient's role during and after catheter insertion.

You should also be prepared to discuss resulting limitations to move-

ment and subsequent management of the infusion site. Review the patient-teaching checklist below before central venous catheter insertion to be sure you have prepared your patient adequately for this procedure.

Patient teaching checklist for central venous catheter insertion

- Assess the patient's knowledge of central venous therapy.
- Reinforce previous explanations of purpose and goal of therapy.
- Tell the patient what to expect during catheter insertion:
–Explain that he will lie in the Trendelenburg position during the procedure with a rolled towel or blanket between his shoulders.
–Tell him a mask will be slipped over his nose and mouth and drapes will cover his body.
–Warn him to expect a stinging sensation during injection of the local anesthetic and pressure during the procedure.
–Explain the suturing procedure.
–Tell the patient which symptoms are important to report.
–Teach the patient how to perform the Valsalva maneuver (patient should return the demonstration).
- Once the catheter is in place:
–discuss physical limitations.
–inform patient about frequency of dressing changes.
–review important symptoms to report (pain, pressure, shortness of breath, or lightheadedness).
–warn the patient to immediately report wet or loose dressings, disconnected tubing, or dislodged catheter.

(*Text continues on page 122.*)

COMPARING CENTRAL VENOUS INFUSION DEVICES

Many different central venous infusion devices are now available. This chart includes a sampling of different catheter types, indications for their use, and special nursing considerations when caring for a patient with a central venous infusion device. Always remember to review your institution's policies and procedures for caring for patients with these devices.

TYPE

Short-term catheters

Single lumen catheter

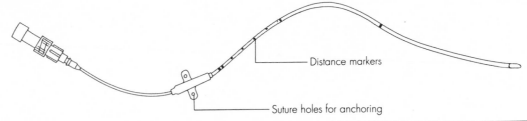

Multiple lumen catheter

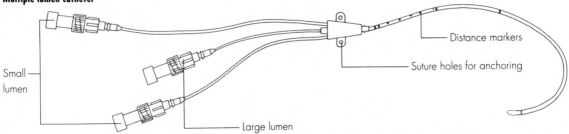

Long-term catheters

Groshong catheter

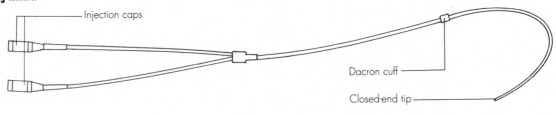

Triple lumen Hickman catheter

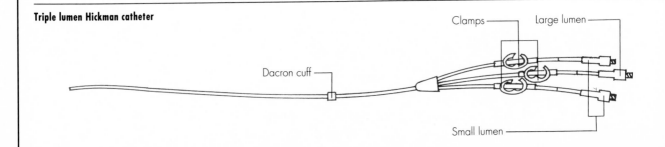

DESCRIPTION	INDICATIONS	NURSING CONSIDERATIONS
• Polyvinyl chloride or polyurethane • Approximately 8" (20.3 cm) long • Lumen gauge varies	• Short-term central venous access • Emergency access • Single purpose therapy: I.V. therapy, antibiotics, total parenteral nutrition (TPN), blood transfusions, chemotherapy • Central venous pressure (CVP) monitoring • Blood sampling for diagnostic testing	• Use sterile technique when caring for insertion site. • Assess frequently for signs of infection and clot formation. • Air elimination filtration may be needed to minimize risk of air emboli formation. • Obtain a chest X-ray to verify catheter placement after insertion.
• Polyvinyl chloride or polyurethane • Double, triple, or quadruple lumens, exiting at 5" (12.7 cm) intervals • Lumen gauge varies • Usually has color-coded lumen ports	• Short-term central venous access • Emergency access • Patient with multiple central venous infusion needs • Patient with limited venous access sites who requires simultaneous multiple infusions that may not be compatible • CVP monitoring • Blood sampling for diagnostic tests.	• Realize that nursing considerations for short-term catheters apply. • Know gauge and purpose of each lumen. • Use the same lumen for the same task. • Remember to label the lumen used for each task. • Heparinize ports not in use to prevent clotting, according to institution policy.
• Silicone rubber • Approximately 35" (88.9 cm) long • Closed end with pressure-sensitive two-way valve • Polyester fiber (Dacron) cuff • Single or multiple lumen	• Long-term central venous access • Heparin allergy • Infusion of I.V. fluids, antibiotics, TPN, blood, and chemotherapy • Blood sampling for diagnostic testing	• Dress the two surgical sites immediately after insertion. • Use a gauze dressing until drainage stops, then use a transparent dressing. • Handle catheter gently because silicone tears easily. • Have catheter repair kit readily available. • Check catheter for kinks or leakage of fluid. • Flush with enough saline to clear length of catheter (especially after blood sampling or blood administration). • Encourage the patient to participate in the care and use of this device as soon as he is able.
• Silicone rubber • Approximately 35" long • Open ended with clamp • Polyester fiber (Dacron) cuff • Single or multiple lumen	• Long-term central venous access • Home I.V. therapy • Infusion of I.V. fluids, antibiotics, TPN, blood, and chemotherapy • Blood sampling for diagnostic testing	• Handle catheter gently and check frequently for kinks, leakage, or tears. • Clamp catheter if it is open or becomes disconnected (use clamp without "teeth"). • Heparinize unused ports according to institution policy. • Encourage the patient to participate in the care and use of device as soon as he is able.

continued

COMPARING CENTRAL VENOUS INFUSION DEVICES *continued*

TYPE

Long-term catheters *continued*

Broviac catheter

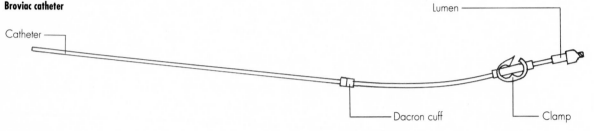

Peripherally inserted central catheter (PICC)

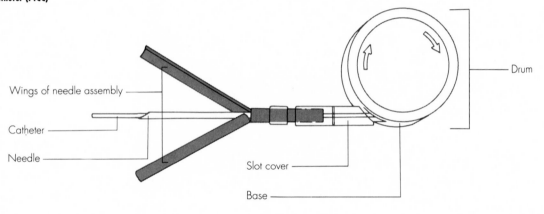

Implantable access device

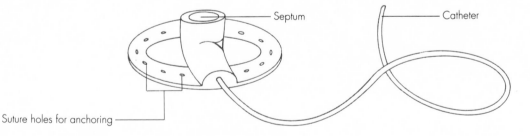

DESCRIPTION	INDICATIONS	NURSING CONSIDERATIONS
• Identical to Hickman except smaller diameter.	• Long-term central venous access • Patients with small central vessels, especially children and elderly patients • Infusion of I.V. fluids, antibiotics, TPN, blood, and chemotherapy • Blood sampling for diagnostic testing	• Handle catheter gently and check frequently for kinks, leakage, or tears. • Clamp catheter if it is open or becomes disconnected (use clamps without "teeth"); clamp eliminates need for Valsalva's maneuver. • Heparinize unused ports according to institution policy. • Encourage the patient to participate in the care and use of the device as soon as he is able.
• Silicone rubber • Single lumen • 16G to 23G • 13" to 28" (33.0 to 71.1 cm) long	• Long-term central venous access • Poor central access • Patients in whom central access may cause fatal complications, or whose surgical site or injury may interfere with insertion • All types of infusion therapy	• Use sterile technique when caring for catheter insertion site. • Heparinize the PICC line after insertion according to institution policy. • Obtain a chest X-ray to confirm catheter placement before starting an infusion. • Change dressing 24 hours after insertion, then every 7 days (more frequently if the dressing becomes wet, loose, or soiled). • Avoid stretching the catheter during dressing changes. • Don't use small diameter tubing for flushing (tuberculin syringe) because it can cause too much pressure; use a 10 ml syringe. • Assess the insertion site, the arm, and the track of the vein for signs of infection. • Instruct the patient on the care of the PICC line.
• Totally implanted port with self-sealing septum attached to a silicone rubber catheter that terminates in the superior vena cava or other body cavity	• Long-term central venous access • Home I.V. therapy • Chemotherapy • Blood sampling for diagnostic tests	• May be difficult to palpate port when entering system (especially if patient is obese). • Leave capped extension tubing and Huber needle in place for repeated injections. • Requires once monthly heparin flush between treatments; dressing changes not required. • Teach patient how to administer medication.

How to assist with central line insertion

1   Begin by verifying the patient's identity and making sure he has signed a consent form. Check the patient's history for hypersensitivity to local anesthetics.

Assemble the necessary equipment. Most institutuions now use preassembled disposable trays with all the necessary supplies including the catheter. If you don't have a pre-assembled tray, you will need the following items: scissors, povidone-iodine solution (Betadine), sterile gauze pads, alcohol, local anesthetic, small syringe with 25G needle, sterile towels or drapes, suture material, suture needle holder, and extra syringes and blood specimen containers if the doctor wishes to draw venous blood samples during catheter insertion.

If your patient's male, check to see if his chest hair covers the intended venipuncture site. If it does, clip the hair close to the skin in an area about 5" (12.7 cm) around the site, then rinse the skin with saline. (Avoid shaving the site because of potential skin irritation). If the patient can tolerate it, place him in the Trendelenburg position. This position encourages the vein to dilate and fill, reducing the risk of air embolism.

2   The doctor usually inserts the catheter on the right side because anatomically the central veins on the right side provide a more direct pathway to the superior vena cava. To position the patient, place a rolled towel or blanket lengthwise between his shoulders, as shown here, to further encourage vein distention. Then place a bedsaver pad under the extremity to prevent blood leakage

onto the bed. Now, to minimize site contamination and make the vein more accessible, turn the patient's head away from the site. Your institution may advocate slipping a mask over the patient's nose and mouth. Explain to him why it's necessary. Don't apply the mask if the patient has difficulty breathing.

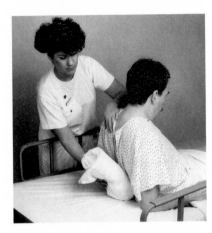

3   Paint the site with povidone-iodine, as shown, and let it air dry for at least 2 minutes. Then repeat this procedure two more times.

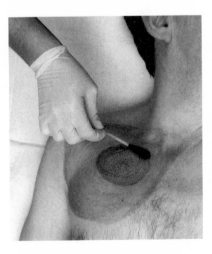

Surround the site with sterile drapes. Have sterile gloves and gown ready for the doctor.

4   Wipe the top of the anesthetic bottle with alcohol. Invert the bottle for the doctor, who'll insert the needle and draw out the solution. The doctor will then inject the local anesthetic into the site, as shown.

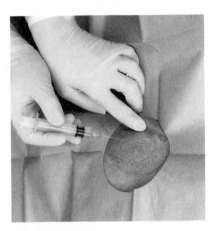

NOTE   The doctor will maintain sterile technique throughout the procedure.

5   If you have not already done so, set up the I.V. solution and administration set while the doctor is anesthetizing the site. This may also be a good time to prepare the infusion pump, if one is being used. See Special Infusion Equipment, page 143, for a discussion of pumps and controllers.

6   The doctor now inserts the needle and catheter as shown.

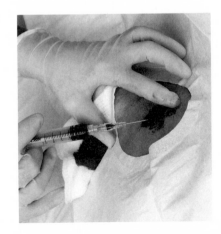

Once the catheter is inserted, the doctor may wish to obtain venous blood samples. If so, this should be done before connecting the fluid-filled I.V. tubing. The nurse is usually responsible for handing the doctor a sterile syringe large enough to hold the amount of blood needed. You will then transfer the blood from the syringe into the proper specimen containers. A vacuum blood specimen tube (Vacutainer) can also be used to obtain blood specimens.

NOTE Current research suggests errors in potassium analysis may result when blood is obtained through a central line because of interfering substances present in the catheter.

7 After the venous blood samples have been taken, the doctor will attach the I.V. line to the catheter hub and suture the catheter in place.

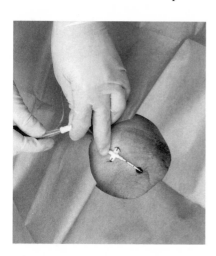

Ask the patient to perform Valsalva's maneuver. This increases intrathoracic pressure, reducing the possibility of air embolus formation. If the subclavian or jugular approach is used, assess the patient's respiratory status for symptoms of distress such as dyspnea, shortness of breath,

and sudden chest pain. Also monitor cardiac status because of the potential for arrhythmias caused by catheter insertion.

At this time, the nurse may set the flow rate of an isotonic I.V. solution at no greater than 20 ml/hour until catheter placement has been confirmed by X-ray.

8 Clean the site with saline to remove any dried blood. Then clean it again with povidone-iodine solution. Place a drop of antibiotic ointment, if policy requires, at the site and cover it with a dry sterile gauze and nonporous tape or a transparent semipermeable dressing.

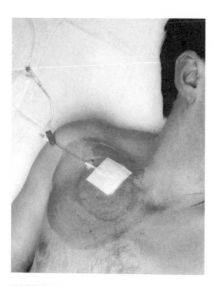

NOTE Keep the patient's head turned away from the site while you apply the dressing.

9 Place the patient in high Fowler's position so he can be X-rayed to confirm catheter placement. If improperly placed, a catheter can cause pneumothorax or cardiac tamponade (see *Central venous line complications*, pages 124 to 126).

If the X-ray shows improper placement, the doctor will adjust the

catheter's position or withdraw it and repeat the procedure. If the catheter position is correct, start the infusion at the prescribed rate.

10 If the tubing you are using does not have locking mechanisms at connection sites, secure all connections with adhesive tape to prevent accidental tube separation, air embolism, or blood loss. Anchor the filter to minimize catheter tension.

11 Now label the dressing with the following: date and time of catheter insertion, the initials of the doctor who inserted it, and the date the dressing was applied. Document all relevant information. Include the type of catheter used, the insertion site, the position of the catheter tip (as seen on X-ray), the distance in centimeters of catheter insertion, the patient's tolerance of the procedure, and if blood samples were collected and sent to the laboratory.

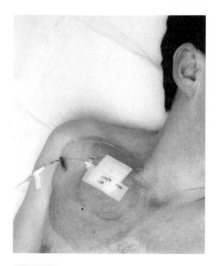

NOTE If the patient has a neck wound or a tracheostomy, place a 3" × 5" sterile drape over the subclavian dressing to protect it from contamination.

(Text continues on page 127.)

CENTRAL VENOUS LINE COMPLICATIONS

SIGNS AND SYMPTOMS	POSSIBLE CAUSES	NURSING ACTIONS	PREVENTION MEASURES

Pneumothorax (accumulation of air or gas in the pleural space), **hemothorax** (collection of blood in the pleural cavity), **chylothorax** (presence of chyle in the thoracic cavity), **hydrothorax** (collection of watery fluid in the pleural cavity)

SIGNS AND SYMPTOMS	POSSIBLE CAUSES	NURSING ACTIONS	PREVENTION MEASURES
• Chest pain • Dyspnea • Cyanosis • Decreased breath sounds • With hemothorax, decreased hemoglobin because of blood pooling • Abnormal chest X-ray	• Puncture of lung with catheter during insertion or exchange over a wire • Puncture of large blood vessel with bleeding inside or outside of lung • Puncture of lymph nodes with leakage of lymph fluid • Infusion of solution into chest area through infiltrated catheter	• Notify doctor. • Remove catheter or assist with removal. • Administer oxygen as ordered. • Set up for and assist with chest tube insertion. • Document your actions.	• Place patient in the Trendelenburg position with a towel roll between the shoulder blades to dilate and expose the vein as much as possible during insertion. • Assess for early signs of fluid infiltration, such as swelling in shoulder, neck, chest, and arm area. • Ensure immobilization of patient via adequate preparation for procedure and restraint during procedure; very active patients may need to be sedated or taken to the operating room for central line insertion.

Air embolism (air in the circulatory system; more common with central lines)

SIGNS AND SYMPTOMS	POSSIBLE CAUSES	NURSING ACTIONS	PREVENTION MEASURES
• Respiratory distress • Unequal breath sounds • Weak pulse • Increased central venous pressure (CVP) • Decreased blood pressure • Churning murmur heard over precordium • Loss of consciousness	• Intake of air into central venous system during catheter insertion or tubing changes; inadvertent opening, cutting, or breakage of catheter	• Clamp the catheter immediately. • Turn patient on left side with head down so air can enter right atrium and be dispersed via pulmonary artery; maintain position for 20 to 30 minutes. • Administer oxygen. • Notify doctor. • Document your actions.	• Purge all air from tubing before hookup. • Teach patient to perform Valsalva's maneuver (see page 127) during catheter insertion and tubing changes. • Use air-eliminating filters proximal to patient. • Use infusion control device with air detection capability. • Use locking tubing, tape connections, or locking devices for all connections.

Blockage of catheter lumen (occluded tip or lumen of catheter inside patient)

SIGNS AND SYMPTOMS	POSSIBLE CAUSES	NURSING ACTIONS	PREVENTION MEASURES
• Inability to flush catheter or infuse fluids without resistance	• Long-term catheterization • Improper flushing or failure to flush on schedule	• Attempt aspiration of clot (do not force clot). • Notify doctor.	• Flush catheter routinely, maintaining positive pressure on plunger of syringe as needle is withdrawn. • Make sure all connections are securely tightened.

CENTRAL VENOUS LINE COMPLICATIONS *continued*

SIGNS AND SYMPTOMS	POSSIBLE CAUSES	NURSING ACTIONS	PREVENTION MEASURES
Blockage of catheter lumen *continued*			
• Inability to withdraw blood from catheter or elicit backflow of blood • Formation of fibrin sheath on catheter tip (seen on X-ray)	• Increased blood clotting because of patient's hematopoietic status • Infusion of incompatible substances through catheter with resultant precipitate formation in lumen • Improper positioning of catheter in vein or tip of catheter placed against wall of vessel	• If ordered, infuse thrombolytic agents such as streptokinase (Streptase) or urokinase (Abbokinase). • If ordered, remove catheter (may be repositioned in vein with verification by X-ray). • Reposition patient (have him lie on side of catheter insertion, cough, and raise arm on side of insertion, lower head of bed and check for flow). • Document your actions.	• Use infusion pump if necessary to overcome venous pressure. • Assess hematologic status of patient. • Heparin may be added to some infusions, such as total parenteral nutrition solution. • Use in-line 0.22-micron filter for infusions. • Monitor chest X-rays to assess catheter position.
Thrombosis (formation of a thrombus)			
• Edema at puncture site • Erythema • Ipsilateral swelling of arm, neck, and face • Pain along vein • Fever, malaise • Tachycardia	• Sluggish flow rate • Catheter material (some materials such as polyvinyl chloride are more thrombogenic) • Hematopoietic status of patient • Preexisting limb edema • Infusion of irritating solutions • Repeated use of same vein or long-term use • Preexisting cardiovascular disease	• Notify doctor. • Remove catheter if ordered. • Infuse anticoagulant doses of heparin if ordered. • Verify thrombosis with diagnostic studies. • Apply warm wet compresses locally. • Do not use limb on affected side for subsequent venipuncture. • Document your actions.	• Maintain flow through catheter at steady rate with infusion pump, or flush at regular intervals. • Use catheters made of less thrombogenic materials or catheters coated to discourage thrombosis. • Dilute irritating solutions. • Use 0.22-micron filter on line.
Local infection (local contamination of insertion site or exit site for silicone rubber [Silastic] catheters, or infection of subcutaneous tunnel for tunnelled catheters)			
• Redness, warmth, tenderness, or swelling at insertion or exit site • Purulent exudate	• Failure to maintain aseptic technique during insertion or site care • Failure to comply with dressing change protocol	• Monitor temperature frequently. • Culture site. • Redress aseptically. • Apply antibiotic ointment as ordered.	• Maintain strict aseptic technique. • Adhere to dressing change protocols. • Teach patient regarding swimming and bathing (patients with adequate white blood cell counts can do these activities at doctor's discretion).

continued

CENTRAL VENOUS LINE COMPLICATIONS *continued*

SIGNS AND SYMPTOMS	POSSIBLE CAUSES	NURSING ACTIONS	PREVENTION MEASURES
Local infection *continued*			
• Local rash or pustules • Fever, chills, malaise	• Wet or soiled dressing remaining on site • Immunosuppression • Irritated suture line	• Treat systemically with antibiotics or antifungals, depending on culture results and doctor's order. • Remove catheter if ordered. • Document your actions.	• Change dressing immediately if site becomes wet or soiled. • Change dressing more frequently if catheter is located in femoral area or near tracheostomy site. • Complete ostomy care and wound dressings after catheter care.
Systemic infection (septicemia or bacteremia caused by introduction of microorganisms into the circulatory system; **primary:** from catheter itself; **secondary:** seeded to catheter from other source)			
• Fever, chills without other apparent reason • Leukocytosis • Nausea, vomiting • Malaise • Elevated urine glucose level	• Contaminated catheter or infusate • Failure to maintain aseptic technique during solution hookup • Frequent opening of catheter or long-term use of single I.V. access • Immunosuppression	• Culture central and peripheral blood samples; if same organism, catheter is primary source of sepsis and should be removed. • If cultures do not match, but are positive, catheter may be removed or the infection may be treated through the catheter. • Treat patient with antibiotic regimen as ordered. • Send tip of device for culture if removed. • Assess for other sources of infection. • Monitor vital signs closely. • Document your actions.	• Examine fluid container for cloudiness, leaks, and turbidity before infusing. • Monitor urine glucose in patients receiving total parenteral nutrition; if greater than +2, suspect early sepsis. • Use strict sterile technique for hookup and discontinuation of fluids. • Use 0.22-micron filter. • Catheter may be changed frequently to decrease chance of infection. • Disturb catheter as little as possible and maintain closed system. • Teach staff and patient about aseptic technique.
Cardiac tamponade (compression of the heart by accumulation of fluid or blood in the pericardial sac)			
• Pulsus paradoxus • Jugular vein distention • Hypotension • Narrowed pulse pressure • Muffled heart sounds • Chest pain • Diaphoresis • Dyspnea • Tachypnea	• Perforation of heart wall by catheter	• Give oxygen if ordered. • Prepare patient for emergency surgery if ordered. • Monitor patient continuously as ordered. • Keep emergency equipment available. • Document your actions.	• Ensure immobilization of patient for procedure. • Assess for signs of cardiac tamponade. • Monitor chest X-rays to assess catheter position.

TEACHING VALSALVA'S MANEUVER

To increase intrathoracic pressure and reduce the risk of air embolus formation during insertion or removal of a central venous catheter, ask the patient to perform Valsalva's maneuver (forced exhalation against a closed airway). Instruct the patient to take a deep breath and hold it, and then bear down for 10 seconds. Then tell him to exhale and breathe quietly. This maneuver initially raises intrathoracic pressure from its normal level of −3 to −4 mm Hg to levels of 60 mm Hg or higher. It also causes slowing of the pulse, decreased return of blood to the heart, and increased venous pressure.

If the patient can't perform Valsalva's maneuver, or if his condition (such as bradycardia, recent eye surgery, myocardial infarction, respiratory distress, or increased intracranial pressure) precludes its use, then remove the catheter while the patient holds his breath after a deep inspiration, while the patient exhales, or while delivering positive pressure via a manual resuscitation bag.

How to change a central venous line dressing

1 The patient with a central line requires a dressing change at his insertion site every 72 hours, sooner if it becomes loose or wet. Many institutions use preassembled trays that contain all of the equipment needed to perform a dressing change.

If your dressing kit has no plastic disposal bag for the discarded dressing, make sure a wastebasket's nearby before you begin the procedure. If your institution does not use these trays, then gather the following equipment: povidone-iodine solution (Betadine), cotton-tipped applicator, antimicrobial ointment, alcohol, hydrogen peroxide, sterile 4" × 4" gauze pads and adhesive tape or sterile 2" × 2" gauze pad and a transparent semipermeable dressing, sterile gloves and masks, and a receptacle for soiled dressings.

Before you begin, explain to the patient exactly what you're about to do. Maintain strict aseptic technique throughout the procedure, beginning with a thorough hand washing. Be sure to wear gloves.

Check to see if policy requires you and the patient to wear face masks during dressing changes. Explain that masks are necessary to prevent I.V. site contamination. Then, slip your mask on, and place the other loosely over the patient's mouth. *Never* put a mask on a patient who needs oxygen or who has a nasogastric tube in place.

2 Place the patient in a supine position. Turn his head away from the dressing to make the insertion site more accessible and to minimize the risk of contamination. Remove the old dressing, taking care not to disturb the catheter.

3 Examine the site for any signs of infection, such as discharge, inflammation, or soreness. If you suspect infection, culture the drainage, send the labeled specimen to the laboratory, and notify the doctor. Then,

check the catheter to make sure it's positioned correctly.

NURSING TIP Measure the length of the catheter from the insertion point to the catheter hub at each dressing change. This will tell you if the catheter is retracting from or advancing into the vein. Document each measurement and notify the doctor if the length changes.

4 Wash your hands, put on another pair of sterile gloves, and clean around the insertion site with an alcohol-soaked cotton-tipped applicator. Work in a circular motion, from the site outward. Take care not to jostle the catheter, or you'll increase the risk of infection.

Do not use acetone because it will have a corrosive effect on the catheter.

5 Clean the site with povidone-iodine as shown, using the circular motion already described. Let the povidone-iodine air dry. Don't use your hands to fan the site. Doing so will increase the risk of contamination. Clean an area approximately the size of the dressing.

Repeat cleaning with povidone-iodine two more times.

6 If policy allows, apply antimicrobial ointment to the insertion site. If the catheter was taped in place, check the tape and replace it if it's soiled. Then cover the catheter site and suture ring with a sterile 4" × 4" gauze pad and secure it with adhesive tape, or place a sterile 2" × 2" gauze pad over the site and apply a large transparent semipermeable dressing.

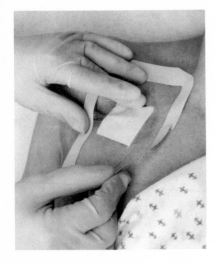

Document your actions in your nurse's notes. Remember to note the catheter measurement and the condition of the insertion site.

How to change central venous line tubing

When a patient receives total parenteral nutrition, you should change the tubing at least every 48 hours, as recommended by the Centers for Disease Control. To do this properly, follow these instructions. Remember to use aseptic technique throughout the procedure, and always wear gloves to reduce your risk of exposure to body fluids. You may also be required to wear a sterile mask. Review institution policy before beginning this procedure.

1 Place a 2" × 2" sterile gauze pad under the catheter connection to create a sterile field. Then clamp the slide clamp on the catheter lumen. Check the connection. If it's very snug, use a hemostat to loosen it before you try to disconnect the tube.

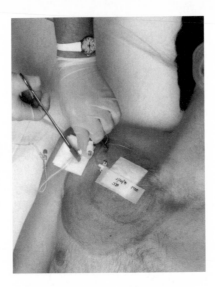

Don't apply too much pressure or you'll crack the hub. If you do, notify the doctor. He'll decide whether or not the catheter should be replaced.

2 Instruct your patient to lie flat. Ask him to perform the Valsalva maneuver (closing his mouth and bearing down)to create internal pressure, making air embolism less likely.

3 Quickly rotate the tubing until it detaches from the hub. Discard it.

4 Insert the new primed tubing into the hub, making sure it's secure (use luer lock tubing when possible).

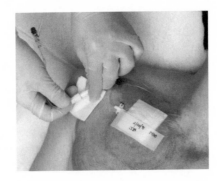

Then, unclamp the slide clamp on the new tubing as shown. Finally, secure all tubing connections with adhesive tape to prevent accidental separation. Document your actions.

How to remove a central line

Long-term central venous catheters and implantable devices are always removed by doctors, usually under surgical conditions. Peripherally inserted central catheters may be removed by qualified RNs. However, nursing responsibilities vary among institutions. Check your institution's policy to see if removal of central lines is a nursing responsibility.

1 Wash your hands and assemble the following equipment: alcohol, povidone-iodine solution (Betadine), sterile gauze pads, tape, forceps or suture removal scissors, sterile gloves, and antimicrobial ointment.

If the tip of the catheter is to be sent for culture, you will also need a sterile specimen container and an extra pair of sterile scissors. Masks will be required for you and the patient.

Review the patient's record for recent reports of catheter placement and catheter length. Explain to the patient what you're about to do.

2 If possible, place the patient in a supine or slight Trendelenburg position. Remove the old dressing (see How to Change a Central Venous Line Dressing). Tell him that he will need to perform the Valsalva maneuver when the catheter is withdrawn and review the maneuver with him if necessary. (Performing this maneuver increases intrathoracic pressure, thus decreasing the risk of air embolus formation.)

3 Put on a pair of sterile gloves and clean the site first with alcohol, then with povidone-iodine solution. Inspect the site for drainage or inflammation. If you suspect infection, culture any drainage from the wound.

> **Take care to avoid cutting the catheter when you remove the sutures.**

Remove the sutures securing the catheter, as shown.

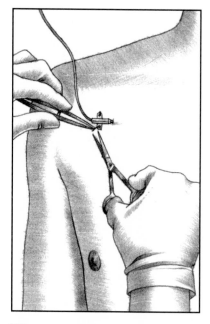

4 Working slowly and carefully, have the patient perform the Valsalva maneuver, and withdraw the catheter from the vein in a slow, even motion.

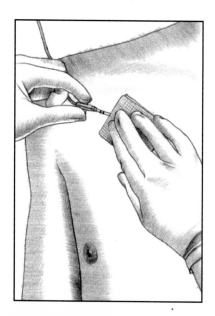

Immediately apply antimicrobial ointment to the insertion site to seal it. Using a 2" × 2" sterile gauze pad or an occlusive dressing, apply manual pressure over the site for 1 minute.

NOTE If the catheter's in a femoral vein, apply manual pressure for at least 5 minutes.

5 Inspect the catheter closely to be sure it's undamaged.

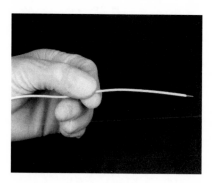

If it's ragged or damaged, notify the doctor immediately. A catheter embolus may be present. Because a damaged catheter may trigger an infection, have the catheter tip cultured, as recommended by the Centers for Disease Control (see How to Remove a Catheter Tip for Culture).

6 Apply antimicrobial ointment and a pressure bandage or occlusive dressing. This prevents air leakage into the vascular system.

7 After 1 hour, remove the pressure bandage and dressing, and apply more antimicrobial ointment. Cover the site with an adhesive bandage strip. Tape the edges down to prevent air leakage into the catheter tract. Instruct the patient to remove this dressing in 24 to 72 hours.

8 Document what you've done in your nurse's notes and in the patient's care plan. Include the date and time of the procedure, the catheter's condition at the time of removal, and the condition of the insertion site. Also note the type of dressing and ointment applied. If you sent the catheter tip or a drainage specimen to the laboratory for culture, include that information too.

How to remove a catheter tip for culture

If a central line-related sepsis is suspected, the doctor will order a culture of the catheter tip. The tip culture is obtained upon removal of the central venous catheter. If removal of a central line is a nursing responsibility at your institution, see How to Remove a Central Line. To obtain a specimen of the catheter tip, follow these steps:

1 Wash your hands and assemble the following equipment: alcohol pads, povidone-iodine solution (Betadine), sterile gloves, two masks, sterile scissors, and a sterile culture container.

2 Explain to your patient exactly what you are about to do. Place a mask on yourself and on the patient to prevent contamination of the catheter site. Then remove the dressing.

3 Clean the site around the central venous catheter with an alcohol pad followed by povidone-iodine solution. Remember to maintain strict aseptic technique during this procedure.

4 After removing the central venous catheter, use sterile scissors to cut a 2" (5.1 cm) segment from the tip of the catheter, as shown.

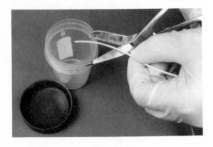

Then place the specimen in the sterile culture container, and label the container appropriately. Send the specimen to the laboratory immediately. Be sure to document your actions in your nurse's notes.

Learning about the peripherally inserted central catheter

Peripherally inserted central catheters (PICC lines) are commonly used for patients receiving home I.V. therapy. These catheters are made of new materials in new designs.

PICC lines are currently available from several manufacturers. They are made of biocompatible silicone elastomer or silicone rubber (Silastic) and polyurethanes. Their small diameters make them easy to insert and comfortable for patients. PICC lines are usually preferred over centrally inserted lines when:
• chest injury is present.
• chest, neck, or shoulder burns are present.
• respiratory function is compromised.
• the surgical site interferes with central catheter placement.
• a doctor is unavailable to insert a central line.

Insertion of a PICC line requires good quality antecubital veins. If these veins have been used for multiple infusions or frequent laboratory sticks, they may be sclerosed and unsuitable for use. The cephalic and basilic veins are used for peripheral insertion of central venous catheters. They both merge into the axillary vein which then becomes the subclavian vein which feeds into the superior vena cava (see *Measuring the peripheral catheter*).

Types of PICC lines

Sooner or later, you will administer I.V. therapy to a patient with a PICC line. The illustration at right will help you become familiar with this type of catheter.

A drum catheter (shown on page 133) is a special silicone catheter for peripheral central venous access. This catheter is elastic and highly flexible. It's wound on a crankcase spool to make insertion easier.

Other more commonly used types of PICC lines consist of a single-lumen silicone elastomer catheter and an introducer needle either with a guide wire or without, as shown. Double-lumen silicone elastomer catheters are also available.

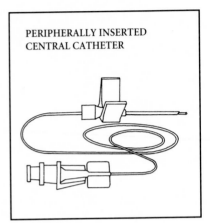

PERIPHERALLY INSERTED CENTRAL CATHETER

P.I.C.C. LINES: ADVANTAGES AND DISADVANTAGES

PICC lines have several benefits as compared to long-term central venous catheters. They are simpler to insert, less expensive, don't require surgery, and are easier for patients to care for at home. The catheter can remain in place for up to 3 months. A PICC line can be used to administer all types of I.V. therapy including parenteral nutrition, antibiotics, blood products, hydrating fluids, and chemotherapy. PICC lines with small lumens are not recommended for obtaining blood samples, as the catheter tends to collapse during aspiration.

Major disadvantages of PICCs are daily care requirements and their effect on activity and body image. The catheter may or may not be sutured in place where it exits the antecubital space, so meticulous care is required to prevent dislodgement. PICC lines can also cause the following complications:
• *Occlusion*. A common risk, which can be reduced by flushing the peripheral line with dilute streptokinase (Streptase), a thrombolytic enzyme.
• *Phlebitis*. Also a common risk but not always a serious one. If the patient receives prompt treatment, you may be able to leave the catheter in place.
• *Infection*. Usually evidenced by purulent drainage at the insertion site, accompanied by an elevated white blood cell count. If you suspect an infection, culture the site. The doctor may want to order an antibiotic and, in severe cases, removal of the line.
• *Catheter sensitivity*. Evidenced by fever and sometimes phlebitis. Usually, the doctor will let the reaction run its course without removing the line. Applying warm compresses to the upper arm often reduces localized phlebitis within 2 days. But if the patient's body continues to resist the catheter, the doctor may order the removal of the line.

PICC lines are usually 20" to 25" (50.8 to 63.5 cm) long, ranging in size from 16G to 23G.

How to insert a PICC line

To insert a PICC line, follow these step-by-step instructions. But remember, you should not try to insert this type of catheter until you've completed formal training as required by institution policy. You should also contact your state board of nursing to find out if you are allowed to insert PICC lines.

1 Explain to the patient exactly what you are about to do. Encourage questions and answer them clearly and honestly. Ensure the patient has signed a consent form, then wash your hands and assemble the necessary equipment. Many manufacturers supply a PICC line tray with all the equipment needed for insertion; the tray below contains a break-away introducer needle, a transparent dressing, povidone-iodine swabsticks, a fenestrated drape with tape, a plain drape, a tape measure, forceps, scissors, alcohol pads, skin protectant, and a poly-lined drape. Also included (but not shown) are a Silastic radiopaque catheter, 2" × 2" gauze pads, sterile cups, a syringe with 18G needle, and povidone ointment.

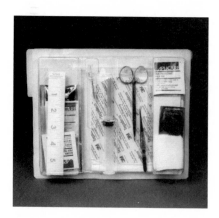

2 Begin with the patient in the supine position with his arm extended laterally to shoulder level. Then, apply a tourniquet at least 4" (10.2 cm) above the antecubital fossa and select an appropriate vein. Remember, either the cephalic or basilic vein can be used. The basilic vein is usually preferred because its straighter course allows for easier advancement. After selecting an appropriate vein, release the tourniquet.

3 Determine the length of the catheter for insertion. To do this, use a nonsterile tape measure. For subclavian placement, measure from the insertion site up the arm to the shoulder. Then, measure across to the midclavicular area.

Measure to the sternal notch and down to the third intercostal space for superior vena cava placement.

4 Because insertion procedures vary by product, be sure to follow the manufacturer's instructions. Put on a gown, mask, and goggles if required. Then, open the tray, set up a sterile field, and put on sterile gloves. Prepare and drape the patient's skin and dilate the antecubital veins as shown.

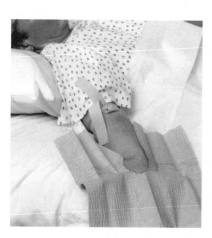

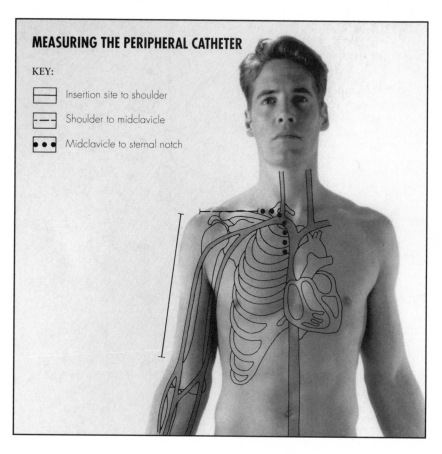

MEASURING THE PERIPHERAL CATHETER

KEY:

Insertion site to shoulder

Shoulder to midclavicle

Midclavicle to sternal notch

THE LANDMARK MIDLINE VENOUS ACCESS DEVICE

The Landmark midline catheter is a new venous access device. This catheter is designed primarily for patients who need I.V. therapy for an intermediate period of time, such as for patients with osteomyelitis who need 4 to 6 weeks of antibiotic therapy, pregnant patients with hyperemesis, or patients with acquired immunodeficiency syndrome who require hydration or antibiotic therapy.

This device is inserted through one of three veins of the antecubital region: the basilic, the cephalic, or the median cubital. However, instead of being advanced into the central venous system, this catheter is threaded only into the veins of the upper arm. Placement in these larger vessels minimizes vein irritation and avoids the risks of infection and pneumothorax usually associated with central venous access. Moreover, this catheter does not require verification by X-ray because the tip is not advanced into the chest veins.

The Landmark midline catheter is made of a bioconforming material called Aquavene. This material is a thromboresistant elastomer hydrogel, which is initially stiff for insertion without a guidewire. Before insertion, this catheter is 6" (15.2 cm) long and is available in either 20G or 22G size. Thirty minutes after contact with body fluid, the catheter softens and expands by two gauge sizes to increase flow capacity, and lengthens by 1" (2.5 cm) to become a 7" (17.8 cm) catheter. The patient's arm must be immobilized for at least 30 minutes after insertion to allow for catheter expansion (see How to Apply Splints and Restraints).

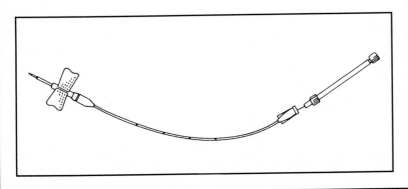

Place a sterile gauze pad over the tourniquet, so you can release the tourniquet without contaminating your sterile gloves.

Using a single-lumen silicone elastomer catheter without a guidewire

1 Use a sterile tape measure from the tray to measure the catheter, adding 1" (2.5 cm) to your earlier measurement. Trim the excess tubing aseptically to the appropriate length according to the manufacturer's recommendations.

2 Attach a 5-ml syringe to the catheter and flush the tubing according to your institution's policy. Leave the syringe attached during the procedure. Then insert the introducer needle with the bevel side up.

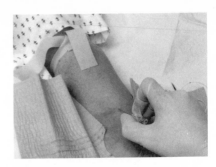

3 Upon entering the vein, expect to see a generous blood return.

4 Using nontoothed forceps, advance the catheter 3" to 4" (7.6 to 10.2 cm) then release the tourniquet. Advance the catheter to the 6" (15.2 cm) mark and have the patient turn his head toward you. Then have him put his chin to his chest to advance the catheter into the subclavian vein.

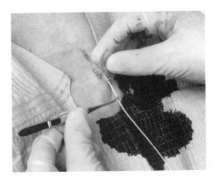

5 Remove the introducer needle from the patient when all but the last few inches of the catheter are in the vein. To remove the needle from the catheter, pinch the wings together (tell the patient she will hear a snap). Cover the site with your other hand to avoid splattering blood.

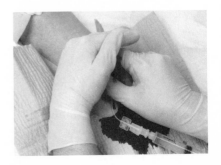

6 Slowly peel the introducer needle apart, stripping the needle cannula away from the catheter.

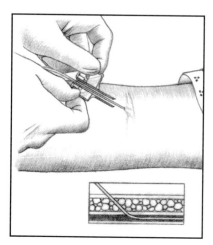

7 Advance the remaining catheter into the vein leaving 1" of the catheter outside the body.

Using a drum catheter

1 Perform the venipuncture, using the indirect method.

2 Turn the crankcase spool counterclockwise to feed the catheter into the vein. Each revolution of the spool feeds approximately 5" (12.7 cm) of the catheter into the vein. Estimate how many revolutions are needed according to your earlier measurement.

3 Continue to feed the catheter into the vein, using the same steps as previously described.

4 When the catheter is inserted, disassemble the crankcase according to the manufacturer's instructions.

When the catheter is in place

1 Check for blood return. Flush the catheter according to your institution's policy and attach the extension tubing to the catheter.

2 Dressing and securing the catheter are two of the most important steps in PICC line insertion. Be sure to secure the catheter according to the manufacturer's recommendations. After securing the catheter and applying a sterile dressing, anchor the extension tubing with tape. Remember that before starting an infusion,

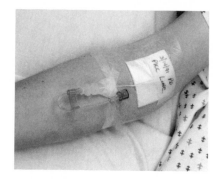

you may need to confirm catheter placement by chest X-ray.

3 Dispose of used equipment appropriately and document your actions.

COMPLICATIONS OF P.I.C.C. LINE INSERTION

Complications can occur at any time during PICC line insertion. You should know how to recognize and treat the following complications:
- bleeding at the insertion site
- cardiac arrhythmias
- catheter embolism
- chest pain
- compartment syndrome
- damage to nerve tissue
- incorrect catheter placement
- respiratory distress
- tendon injury.

Postinsertion complications to watch for include:
- phlebitis
- cellulitis
- catheter sepsis
- thrombosis
- thrombophlebitis
- air embolism
- pulmonary embolism.

Complications of PICC line insertion are best avoided through skillful insertion technique and careful patient screening.

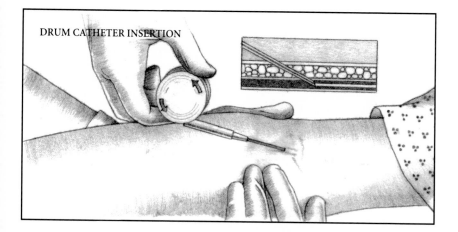

DRUM CATHETER INSERTION

Special Infusion Techniques

Intraosseous infusion

Intraosseous administration may be indicated in a severe emergency in which I.V. access is not readily available for infusing necessary fluids and medications. Such emergencies include cardiopulmonary arrest or circulatory collapse, hypokalemia from trauma or dehydration, status epilepticus, status asthmaticus, burns, near drowning, and overwhelming sepsis. Any drug that can be given intravenously can be given intraosseously, and drug absorption and effectiveness are the same as by the I.V. route. However, use of the intraosseous route is usually limited to very young children because the vascular red marrow is replaced by the less vascular yellow marrow at about age 5.

During intraosseous infusion, the bone marrow serves as a noncollapsible vein; thus, fluid infused into the marrow cavity rapidly enters the systemic circulation via an extensive network of venous sinusoids (see lateral view of tibial intraosseous infusion shown below).

Intraosseous flow rates are determined by both the size of the needle and the flow through the bone marrow. Fluids should flow freely if needle placement is correct. When it is, the needle stands upright without support. Normal saline has been administered intraosseously at a rate of 600 ml/minute and up to 2,500 ml/hour when delivered under pressure of 300 mm Hg through a 13G needle.

Contraindications and precautions

Absolute contraindications to intraosseous infusion include osteogenesis imperfecta, osteopetrosis, and ipsilateral fracture, because of the potential for subcutaneous extravasation. Infusion through an area with cellulitis or an infected burn increases the risk of infection.

Procedure

With specialized training, insertion of a needle for intraosseous infusion can be accomplished within 3 minutes, using the following procedure:

The patient's leg is restrained with a sandbag supporting the knee, and the skin is cleaned aseptically with iodine or alcohol. A local anesthetic may be administered before insertion of the needle, but may be unnecessary in emergency situations when the patient is severely obtunded or unconscious. The optimal site of insertion is the proximal tibia, where placement will not interfere with ventilation or chest compression. An injection site is selected in the midline on the medial flat surface of the anterior tibia two finger widths (1 to 3 cm) below the tibial tuberosity. The needle is directed at a 60- to 90-degree angle, away from the growth plate to avoid damaging it, and is advanced with a screwing motion. After the needle has passed through the cortex, it advances without resistance into the marrow space. Marrow can be aspirated easily into a syringe and fluid infused easily. To prevent clotting during infusion, flushing the needle with heparin-saline solution should precede attachment to an appropriate infusion set.

Complications

During intraosseous infusion, monitor for the most common complications: extravasation of fluid into subcutaneous tissue, resulting from incorrect needle placement; subperiosteal effusion, resulting from failure of fluid to enter the marrow space; and clotting in the needle, resulting from delayed infusion or failure to flush the needle after placement.

Discontinuation

Intraosseous infusion should be discontinued as soon as conventional vascular access is established, within 2 hours if possible. Prolonged infusion significantly increases the risk of a complicating infection.

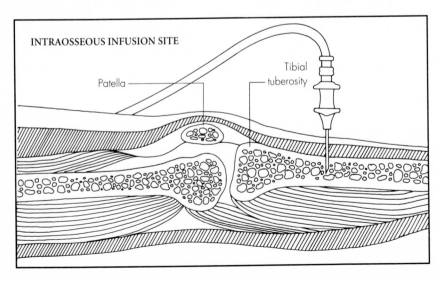

INTRAOSSEOUS INFUSION SITE

Patella

Tibial tuberosity

SITE OF EPIDURAL INFUSION

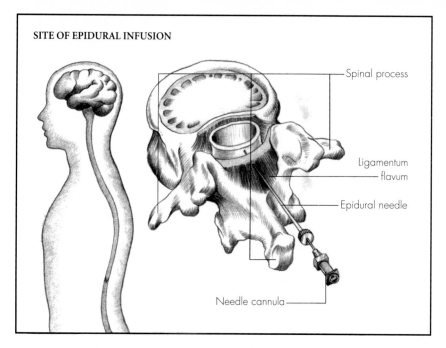

Spinal process

Ligamentum flavum

Epidural needle

Needle cannula

After the needle is withdrawn, a sterile dressing should be applied over the injection site, with firm pressure applied to the dressing for 5 minutes.

Epidural analgesia

The epidural space lies between the dura and the ligamentum flavum, outside the subarachnoid space where cerebrospinal fluid (CSF) flows. A drug injected or infused into this area diffuses slowly into the subarachnoid space and then into the CSF, which carries it directly to the spinal nervous system, bypassing the blood-brain barrier.

Epidural infusions can effectively control both acute and chronic pain, including moderate to severe postop-erative pain. In patients with chronic pain, such as those with cancer, degenerative joint disease, or spinal trauma, epidural analgesia relieves pain without frequent injections or the cumbersome intravenous equipment required by other methods. Continuous epidural infusion of a low concentration opiate analgesic produces excellent pain control in most patients, without the analgesic peaks and valleys associated with intermittent I.M injections. Because epidural administration is associated with minimal central and systemic distribution of the drug, it relieves pain originating anywhere below the cranial nerves with smaller doses and less severe adverse effects. The consistent pain control that an implanted permanent epidural catheter can provide may also allow a shorter hospitalization.

Contraindications to epidural infusion include local or systemic infection, neurologic disease, anticoagulant therapy, coagulopathy, spinal arthritis or deformity, hypotension or marked hypertension, and allergy to the proposed drug. Home use of epidural analgesia is not an option if

COMPARING EPIDURAL ANALGESICS

Morphine is commonly used for epidural infusion because it is relatively inexpensive and produces few tissue reactions. The therapeutic dose range for an epidural infusion of morphine is 0.2 to 2.0 ml/hour. If prepared in a concentration of 10 mg/100 ml of normal saline, the infusion rate would be 2 to 20 ml/hour, or 0.1 mg/ml/hour. If your patient experiences adverse reactions such as nausea, vomiting, pruritus, or respiratory depression, another opiate may be substituted. Be sure, however, that the infusion container of any drug selected is labelled "For epidural use only". Epidural solutions are preservative-free and nontoxic to epidural membranes.

Analgesic	Dose	Onset (minutes)	Peak (minutes)	Duration (hours)
Morphine sulfate	1 to 10 mg	<30	30 to 60	18 to 24
Fentanyl citrate (Sublimaze)	50 to 100 mcg	<10	10 to 15	4 to 6
Hydromorphine hydrochloride (Dilaudid)	0.5 to 3 mg	<10	10 to 20	6 to 17

the patient or his family is unwilling or unable to learn the care needed, or if the patient can't be relied on to refrain from alcohol or street drugs, because these substances potentiate opiate action.

Because it is so effective in managing severe pain, epidural analgesia is becoming more common in some health care settings. It provides adequate, consistent pain relief that increases the patient's trust and facilitates nursing care. To provide such analgesia, specially trained primary nurses now have the authority (depending on state nurse practice acts and individual institution policy) to assess the patient's pain level and administer an analgesic to prevent severe pain.

Setup for epidural analgesia

An epidural catheter is inserted by an anesthesiologist into the low back (T10 to L4) at a site selected according to the region to be affected. The catheter is threaded 1¼" to 2" (3.2 to 5.1 cm) into the epidural space. To check placement of the catheter, the anesthesiologist injects a small bolus of local anesthetic into the catheter. If placement is correct, the injection will have no obvious effect. However, if the catheter was inadvertently placed into the spinal space, the patient will rapidly develop leg numbness. After the needle has been introduced into the spinal space, the cannula is removed and the catheter is inserted.

For temporary analgesic therapy (less than a week), the catheter may exit directly over the spine and be taped up the patient's back to the shoulder. However, for prolonged therapy, the catheter may be tunneled subcutaneously to an exit site on the patient's side or abdomen, as shown.

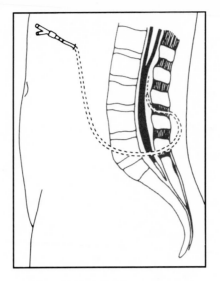

The dressing over the exit site is usually transparent to allow inspec-tion for drainage. The dressing often appears moist or slightly blood tinged. An epidural dressing is usually changed every 24 to 48 hours. Check your institution's policy to see if this dressing change is a nursing responsibility.

An implanted injection port or infusion pump may be attached to the catheter if needed. However, the catheter is usually connected to special epidural infusion tubing, which has no ports to prevent accidental injection of a drug meant for intravenous use. If epidural infusion tubing is not available, all ports and connections should be covered with tape and clearly labeled "Epidural Infusion."

MANAGING ADVERSE EPIDURAL DRUG REACTIONS

The most common complication of epidural infusion is numbness and leg weakness, which is drug and concentration dependent. Identifying the dosage level that provides adequate pain control without causing excessive numbness and weakness requires that the doctor titrate the dosage.

COMMON ANTAGONISTS FOR MANAGING ADVERSE EPIDURAL DRUG REACTIONS

Adverse drug reaction	Agent	Route	Pharmacologic class
Respiratory depression	Naloxone (Narcan) 0.2 to 0.4 mg	I.V.	Narcotic antagonist
Pruritus	Nalbuphine (Nubain) 5 mg	I.V.	Synthetic narcotic agonist-antagonist
	Diphenhydramine (Benadryl) 25 mg	I.V.	Antihistamine
Nausea, vomiting	Prochlorperazine (Compazine) 5 to 10 mg	I.M.	Antiemetic
	Metoclopramide 10 mg	I.M. or I.V.	GI stimulant

Assisting with insertion of an epidural catheter

If you are assisting with an epidural insertion on the unit, you will need to gather the following equipment: a commercially prepared epidural tray similar to the one shown below, epidural infusion tubing, a transparent dressing, 3" (7.6 cm) silk tape to secure the tubing to the back, if necessary, and optional monitoring equipment for blood pressure and pulse rate.

Now, make the following preparations:

• Make sure that a consent form has been properly signed and witnessed.

• Be sure the pharmacy has been notified ahead of time regarding the medication order, as epidural solutions require special preparation.

• Make sure the patient understands the procedure and its possible complications, including the placement of the catheter, its use, and who will administer pain medication. Tell the patient to expect the use of monitors during the immediate postoperative period, and emphasize the importance of reporting pain as soon as he perceives it. To help the patient describe the intensity of his pain, you may use a visual analog pain scale.

• Just before the procedure, position the patient on his side in the knee-chest position or have him sit at the edge of the bed leaning over a bedside table (as shown), depending on the doctor's preference.

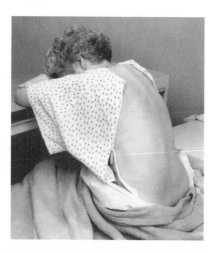

WHAT IS A BLOOD PATCH?

When CSF leaks into the dura mater during insertion of an epidural catheter (called a wet tap), headache usually results. This post-analgesia headache worsens with postural changes such as standing or sitting.

The treatment for such headache is a "blood patch." The patient's own blood (approximately 10 ml) is withdrawn from a peripheral vein and then injected into the epidural space. When the epidural needle is withdrawn, the patient is instructed to sit up. Because the blood clots seal off the leaking area, the blood patch should relieve the patient's headache immediately. The patient need not restrict his activity after this procedure.

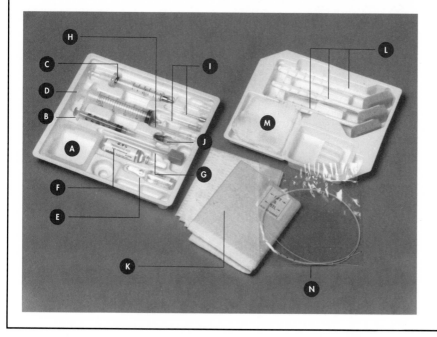

A   Medicine cup
B   3-ml syringe
C   5-ml syringe
D   20-ml syringe
E   Local anesthetic
F   Sodium chloride for injection
G   Epidural needle
H   Filter needle
I   15G and 21G needles
J   Luer adapter
K   Drape
L   Swab sticks
M   Sterile gauze pads
N   Catheter

NURSING CARE PLANS FOR THE PATIENT WITH AN EPIDURAL CATHETER

Because of its location, the potential for migration through the dura, and the proximity to spinal nerves and vessels, use of an epidural catheter is associated with severe complications. Recognizing and preventing such complications are primary concerns in developing a nursing care plan for the patient with an epidural catheter. The chart below includes typical elements of nursing care for such a patient.

NURSING DIAGNOSIS	GOAL	PLAN OR INTERVENTION
Ineffective breathing pattern	To maintain adequate ventilation and perfusion	• Assess rate, depth, and regularity of respiration. Observe chest expansion every hour for 24 hours after infusion. • Auscultate breath sounds every shift and as needed. • Assess SaO_2 via continuous pulse oximetry to maintain SaO_2 above 95%. • Encourage and instruct patient to perform effective deep-breathing and coughing techniques. • Administer naloxone (Narcan) as ordered. • Have manual resuscitation bag with mask suction and oxygen at bedside. • Avoid the use of supplemental opiates, if possible.
Impaired skin integrity	To maintain skin integrity	• Control itching with intermittent applications of cool compresses. • Give antihistamines as ordered. • Explain and emphasize the importance of not scratching. • Keep patient's skin clean and dry. • Carefully titrate the opiate dosage. • Use only preservative-free analgesic solutions.
Altered urinary elimination	To achieve normal pattern of urinary elimination	• Palpate bladder every shift. • Encourage voiding by using measures such as privacy, warm bed pan, running water, male standing, female sitting. • Catheterize as ordered. • Monitor fluid intake and output.
Fluid volume deficit related to nausea or vomiting	To maintain adequate fluid volume	• Administer I.V. fluids as ordered. • Administer antihistamines as ordered, and note their effectiveness. • Plan fluid intake goal for each shift based on intake and output. • To encourage fluid intake, assess the patient's preferences and provide favorite fluids. • Give small amounts of fluid frequently. • Titrate opiate dosage carefully. • Protect patient from aspiration.

NURSING CARE PLANS FOR THE PATIENT WITH AN EPIDURAL CATHETER *continued*

NURSING DIAGNOSIS	GOAL	PLAN OR INTERVENTION
Fluid volume deficit related to CSF leakage	To maintain adequate fluid volume	• Assess any signs and symptoms of headache related to patient's position. • Maintain adequate fluid intake avoiding caffeine and sweetened fluids. • Provide quiet, dark environment. • Keep patient as calm as possible.
Pain	To increase comfort, decrease restlessness, and increase mobility	• Assess and document the severity of pain using a scale of 1 to 10. Ask the patient to indicate the location of the pain and tell if the pain is sharp, dull, constant, or intermittent. • Titrate epidural dosage as ordered and document dosage changes. • Monitor for and document adverse reactions to epidural infusion (respiratory depression, nausea, vomiting, pruritus, urine retention). • Monitor patient's response and notify doctor or anesthesiologist if pain is not controlled. • Assess if pain has become unilateral or if pain relief has changed (breakthrough pain). Report such changes to the anesthesiologist immediately.

Discontinuing epidural analgesic therapy

Normally, the doctor removes the catheter. However, if policy allows a specially trained nurse to remove the catheter, follow these guidelines:

• If you feel resistance when removing the catheter, stop and call the doctor for further orders.

• Be sure to save the catheter because the doctor will want to examine the catheter tip for any shearing during removal.

• Keep in mind that drugs used epidurally diffuse slowly and may cause effects, including excessive sedation, up to 12 hours after epidural infusion has been discontinued.

Documentation

Throughout epidural catheter use, you should document the patient's response to treatment, catheter patency, condition of the dressing and insertion site, vital signs, and assessment results. Also document the labeling of the epidural catheter and changing of the infusion bags, as well as any supplemental analgesic requirements. A flow sheet helps identify trends.

The Ommaya reservoir: Intraventricular access to CSF

Designed to deliver long-term therapy with antibiotics, antifungal agents, analgesics, and chemotherapeutic drugs to the cerebrospinal fluid

(CSF) via the ventricles, the Ommaya reservoir spares the patient repeated lumbar punctures. The most common uses are chemotherapy and pain management. Besides providing convenient, comparatively painless access to CSF, the Ommaya reservoir permits consistent and predictable drug distribution throughout the subarachnoid space and central nervous system and provides a method for measuring intracranial pressure. As the Ommaya reservoir's use becomes more prevalent, you may soon care for a patient who has one.

Before insertion of the reservoir, the patient may receive either a local or general anesthetic, depending on the patient's condition and the doctor's preference. Then the doctor

COMPLICATIONS OF EPIDURAL INFUSION

COMPLICATIONS	POSSIBLE CAUSES	SIGNS AND SYMPTOMS	NURSING INTERVENTION	PREVENTION
Headache	Leakage of CSF	• Increasing headache related to postural changes • Muscle aches • Visual symptoms: double vision, difficulty in focusing, blurred vision, spots • Hearing problems: buzzing, roaring, popping	• Increase fluid intake; decrease caffeine and sugar. • Provide quiet, dimly lit environment. • Before procedure, teach patient about blood patch.	• Instruct the patient to lie flat. • Maintain adequate fluid intake.
Change in analgesic effects	Migration of catheter	• Unilateral analgesic effect • Change in respiration rate • Hypotension • Nausea	• Notify anesthesiologist if respiration rate decreases. • Administer oxygen and I.V. fluids. • Discontinue opiate.	• Securely tape catheter along spinal cord at its exit site. • Monitor hash mark on catheter indicating length.
Redness and swelling at catheter insertion site	Infection	• Fever • Increased white blood cell count • Unusual drainage	• Notify anesthesiologist.	• Change dressings according to hospital policy. • Discard premixed epidural solutions after 48 hours. • Use sterile technique. • Securely tape all connections.

OMMAYA RESERVOIR IMPLANTED BENEATH PATIENT'S SCALP

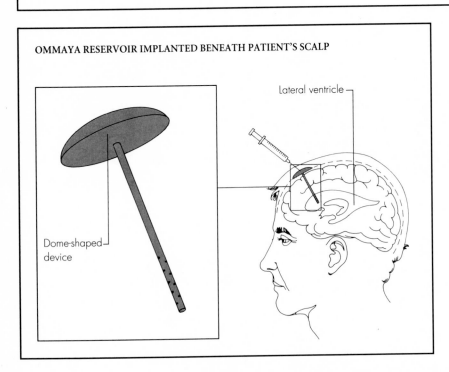

Lateral ventricle

Dome-shaped device

drills a burr hole and inserts the device's catheter through the patient's nondominant frontal lobe into the lateral ventricle as shown. The reservoir, which has a self-sealing silicone injection dome, rests over the burr hole under a scalp flap. This creates a slight, soft bulge on the scalp, approximately the size of a quarter. After an X-ray confirms placement, a pressure dressing is applied for 24 hours, followed by a gauze dressing for another day or two. The sutures may be removed in about 10 days. However, the reservoir can be used within 48 hours to deliver drugs, obtain CSF pressure measurements, drain CSF, and withdraw CSF specimens.

If your patient is scheduled for placement of an Ommaya reservoir, explain the procedure before the reservoir is inserted. Be sure the patient and his family understand the potential complications and answer any questions they may have. Reassure the patient that any hair shaved for the implant will grow back, and that only a coin-sized patch must remain shaved for injections. The patient must protect the site from bumps and trauma while the incision heals, and unless complications develop, the reservoir may function for years.

The outpatient may quickly resume normal activities. However, instruct the patient and his family to notify the doctor if any signs of infection develop at the insertion site (for example, redness, swelling, tenderness, or drainage), or if the patient develops headache, neck stiffness, or fever, which may indicate a generalized infection. Such infections can usually be treated successfully by injection of antibiotics directly into the reservoir. Persistent infection may require the removal of the reservoir.

Another possible complication, catheter migration or blockage, may cause symptoms of increased intracranial pressure, such as headache and nausea. If he suspects this problem, the doctor may gently push and release the reservoir several times (a technique called pumping). With his finger on the patient's scalp, the doctor can feel the reservoir refill. Slow filling suggests catheter migration or blockage, which must be confirmed by computerized tomography scan. Surgical correction is required.

Preparing to access the Ommaya reservoir

The doctor usually instills chemotherapeutic agents or opioids into the Ommaya reservoir, but a specially trained nurse may perform this procedure if institution policy and the state practice act allows. This sterile procedure usually takes 15 to 30 minutes. Equipment varies but usually includes the following: the preservative-free prescribed drug, sterile gloves, povidone-iodine solution (Betadine), 3-ml sterile syringe, 25G sterile needle or a 22G noncoring (Huber) needle, collection tubes for CSF if ordered, and a vial of bacteriostatic saline. Occasionally, the doctor may wish to prescribe an antiemetic to be administered one-half hour before the procedure to control nausea and vomiting.

Accessing the Ommaya reservoir

• Obtain baseline vital signs.
• Assess the patient and his family health history since his last visit (specifically review the history of colds, fevers, headaches, nausea, and vomiting).
• Prepare a syringe with the drug to be instilled and place it, the CSF collection tubes, and the saline solution within reach of the sterile field.
• Position the patient in either a sitting or reclining position.
• Establish a sterile field near the patient and place the needle and syringe on it.
• Put on gloves and prepare the patient's scalp with the povidone-iodine solution, working in a circular motion from the center outward.
• Now, placing the 25G needle at a 45-degree angle, access the reservoir and aspirate 3 ml of clear CSF into a syringe (if you get anything but clear CSF, check with the doctor before continuing).
• Continue to aspirate as many milliliters of CSF as you will instill of the drug. Then detach the syringe from the needle hub, attach the drug syringe, and instill the medication slowly, monitoring for headache, nausea, and dizziness. (Some institutions use the CSF instead of a preservative-free diluent to deliver the drug).

• Follow institution policy regarding reinstilling the CSF you withdrew and completing the procedure with a 2 to 3 ml saline flush.
• Instruct the patient to lie quietly for approximately 15 to 30 minutes after the procedure. This may prevent meningeal irritation leading to nausea and vomiting.

Post-access care

• Cover the site with a sterile gauze pad and apply gentle pressure for a moment or two until superficial bleeding stops.
• Monitor the patient for signs of increased intracranial pressure, such as nausea, vomiting, pain, or dizziness, and drug effects. Assess for these effects every 30 minutes for 2 hours, then every hour for 2 hours, and finally every 4 hours.
• Documentation should include the appearance of the site before and after access, the patient's tolerance of the procedure, how much CSF was withdrawn and the name and dose of the drug instilled.

Intraperitoneal therapy

Intraperitoneal (IP) therapy, the administration of a therapeutic agent directly into the peritoneal cavity, has become more common, mainly as a result of its usefulness in cancer research. The rationale for IP administration is the goal of increasing concentration of the antineoplastic agents at the tumor site (peritoneal cavity) to enhance the drug's penetration and cytotoxic effects while limiting systemic effects. IP administration allows peak drug levels at the tumor site far beyond those that could be tolerated systemically.

IP therapy is effective in treating carcinomas of the ovaries and fallopian tubes. It is also being used to treat colorectal, endometrial, gastric, bladder, and breast cancers and other cancers of unknown origin.

INTRAPERITONEAL ACCESS DEVICES

The most common IP access devices are listed below with their related advantages and disadvantages.

I.P. ACCESS DEVICE	ADVANTAGES	DISADVANTAGES
Temporary indwelling catheter (percutaneous placement)	• May be inserted at the bedside. • Doesn't require surgical removal. • Catheter is inexpensive. • Temporary presence decreases the risk of infection and fibrous sheath formation. • Doesn't require home care.	• Percutaneous insertion increases risk of bowel or visceral perforation. (As a temporary catheter, it is not usually recommended for cyclic therapy because of the need for repeated placement.) • Repeated puncture and drug instillation increase the risk of perforating the bowel or a vessel, especially if it is fibrosed to the peritoneal surface. • Requires extra precautions to prevent displacement when mobilizing patient.
Implantable port	• Serves as a semipermanent access device and allows for long-term cyclic treatments. • Decreases risk of bowel or visceral perforation when inserted during laparotomy. • Doesn't require catheter home care (no external catheter). • Implantable system decreases the risk of infection under less than ideal conditions. • Absence of an external catheter improves patient acceptance.	• Requires surgical insertion. • Requires surgical procedure for removal. • Is an expensive access device. • Doesn't allow for high-pressure (> 40 psi), forced irrigation or manipulation to dislodge or loosen fibrin clots. • Each access requires a needle stick.
Indwelling catheter	• Serves as a semipermanent access device and allows long-term cyclic treatments. • Decreases risk of bowel or visceral perforation when inserted during laparotomy. • Is an inexpensive catheter. • Allows for high-pressure, forced irrigation and manipulation to dislodge or loosen fibrin clots. • Permits rapid instillation of fluid (2 liters over 10 to 15 minutes). • Permits rapid drainage of peritoneal fluid in absence of occlusion. • Requires pulling to remove, no surgical incision. • May be preferred in an obese patient.	• Requires surgical insertion. • External catheter component increases risk of infection, especially under less than ideal conditions. • External catheter requires home care. • External catheter may create body image changes.

Special Infusion Equipment

Pumps and controllers: Electronic infusion devices

When you need to monitor an intravenous infusion, you'll probably use one of the many electronic infusion devices now available. Here's an overview of what they are, how they differ, and how they can help.

Electronic control devices are classified as either infusion controllers or infusion pumps. Both permit accurate, on time delivery of fluids and drugs. They allow immediate adjustment of inflow rates, decrease the number of hands-on infusion checks, prevent too rapid infusion, reduce the incidence of infiltration, and maintain patency of the cannula.

Guidelines for use of infusion pumps and controllers vary depending on institution policy. They may be used to administer certain drugs, especially aminophylline, heparin, fibrinolytic agents, high-dose potassium chloride, vasopressors, antiarrhythmics, insulin, and antineoplastic drugs. Other uses include total parenteral nutrition, infusions delivered through a central line, infusions for patients on fluid restriction, drug infusions for infants and children under age 7, and infusions for patients with limited venous access. Either type may require special cassette tubing or use standard I.V. tubing.

What's the difference between a controller and a pump?

The primary difference is that a pump can add pressure to the infusion to overcome resistance to the flow, but a controller can't. The maximum flow rate with a controller depends on how high you hang the I.V. container above the I.V.

ELECTRONIC INFUSION DEVICE FEATURES

Pumps and controllers include the following settings:

- power on and off
- infusion rate
- infusion volume
- stop and start (power remains on)
- alarm silence
- battery operation (time limit varies with the machine)
- indicator flow light.

Additional features may include:

- keep-open rate when preset volume is infused
- panel light
- tamper-proof lock
- runaway prevention
- infiltration detection
- lock-out mechanisms
- nurse call-light integration
- panel lights
- flow status monitors.

Dual chamber pumps are also available, such as the Flo-Gard 6300. Some pumps can deliver up to 10 infusions, piggybacks, or I.V. push drugs.

Both types may have alarms that are activated by:

- occlusion
- air in line
- completed infusion
- open pump door.

The following pages will discuss how to use the Flo-Gard 6300 volumetric infusion pump and the "Plum" Life-Care 5000 drug delivery system.

---

site. Hanging an I.V. bag 36" (90 cm) above a patient's head while he is lying flat will provide adequate gravity pressure for the I.V. flow. The controller will then ensure delivery of a set amount of fluid over a certain period of time. When there is resistance to the flow, for example, because of occlusion in the I.V. system or increased vascular backflow, the controller's alarm will sound, signaling that it can't maintain the preset I.V. rate. Because resistance can occur when the patient moves, this alarm can sound often. Some controllers have indicator lights that signal a need to check the I.V. site and correct a resistance problem before the alarm sounds.

An infusion pump controls the flow rate totally. If gravity pressure does not deliver the infusion at a preset rate, the pump adds a driving pressure to the system. The amount of pressure measured in pounds per square inch (psi) determines how much resistance the pump can overcome. But the pump will not exceed preset limits. When the pump exerts maximum preset pressure (occlusion pressure), the machine's alarm sounds and the infusion stops. New pump models do not exceed 15 psi, which is considered a safe limit. However, some pumps include an optional setting called "variable pressure" that allows the nurse to set the pressure limit. Because of their greater accuracy in delivering the infusion and fewer nuisance alarms if the patient is active, many clinicians prefer pumps to controllers.

The common fear that driving pressure generated by pumps causes infiltration is unfounded. However, if infiltration occurs, the pump will

UNDERSTANDING I.V. RESISTANCE

Infusion of fluid into the veins must overcome resistance caused by the I.V. delivery system and the pressure created by the patient's blood flow.

• *Resistance in the I.V. system* can result from lumen bore (size) of the tubing, fluid viscosity, catheter gauge, or kinked tubing or blocked catheters. I.V. filters cause little resistance because they have a broad surface capacity. But smaller (micron size) microaggregate blood filters may reduce the blood flow of packed cells because of the cells' viscosity.

• *Increased vascular resistance* can result from thrombosed, narrowed, or scarred veins. This contributes to vascular back pressure or backflow of the I.V.

Gravity pressure (70 mm Hg or 1.3 psi) is usually sufficient for infusing most fluids. Gravity pressure is reached by placing the I.V. solution at least 36" (90 cm) above the patient's vein. Because peripheral or central line venous back pressure is usually 30 to 50 mm Hg, gravity pressure can overcome it.

When viscous solutions or high venous back pressures are encountered, the resistance pressure in the vein can increase to 100 to 150 mm Hg (2 to 3 psi). If this happens or if the patient has arterial lines with a vascular pressure of 300 mm Hg (6 psi), you'll need to use a pump instead of a controller to overcome the higher pressures.

Coughing, straining, crying, walking, sitting, and standing can significantly increase back pressure. This is particularly noticeable in young, relatively healthy patients.

FLO-GARD 6300

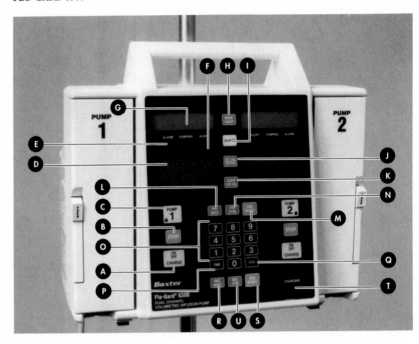

A On-off and charge key	**H** Backlight key	**O** Numerical keyboard
B Stop key	**I** Silence key	**P** Time key
C Pump 1 key and indicator	**J** Total volume and status key	**Q** Clear key
D Pump 1 main display	**K** Clear total volume key	**R** Secondary rate key
E Pump 1 alarm light	**L** Primary rate key	**S** Secondary start key
F Pump 1 alert light	**M** Primary start key	**T** Charging light
G Pump 1 message display	**N** Primary volume to be infused key	**U** Secondary volume to be infused key

continue the infusion, which could make the infiltration worse. So, remember to monitor the I.V. site carefully when using an electronic control device.

Learning about the Flo-Gard 6300 pump

Your patient is receiving several intravenous medications. Throughout your shift, you administer antibiotics every 4 hours, monitor intravenous infusions, and frequently check I.V. lines for patency. Imagine how much time you'd save if a pump could take over some of these functions.

The Flo-Gard 6300, a dual channel volumetric infusion pump, can perform these functions and more. This state-of-the-art equipment will greatly reduce your work load and increase your patient's safety.

Pump design and function

Designed to perform the functions of two conventional pumps, the Flo-Gard 6300 runs on wall power or battery power for up to 6 hours with one pump running and up to 43 hours with both pumps running at rates from 1 to 1,400 ml/hour. Each pump uses a standard Baxter solution

I.V. SET LOADING

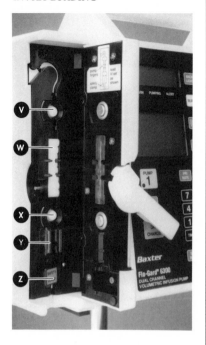

V Upstream occlusion sensor
W Pump mechanism
X Downstream occlusion sensor
Y Air sensor
Z Safety clamp

administration set and features an independent secondary medication program for intermittent infusions. However, when performing automatic piggybacking, use a Baxter Continu-Flo solution set as the primary set.

This 17.6 lb pump, shown above, can be attached to a standard I.V. pole. The pump's front panel displays controls and indicators associated with each channel.

The adjacent photo shows the loading mechanism of pump 1 with the door open. Pump 2 has identical features.

Safety features

Whenever it's turned on, the pump performs an automatic self-test of electrical and mechanical components. It maintains a 5-hour memory of infusion data after the power is off. You can't accidentally change programmed information, because each change would require additional entries (see How to Program the Flo-Gard Primary Line, page 146). The device's front panel can be locked during pumping to prevent tampering. An additional safety device is the volume-time programming that automatically calculates the required flow rate.

Problems or changes anywhere in the system activate the pump's audible alarm and visual message display. The display screen indicates the problem, but you must determine the cause and intervene appropriately

How to set up the Flo-Gard 6300 pump

Before using the pump, refer to the manufacturer's operations manual. The manual also provides instructions for special pump functions.

1 Clamp the pump securely to an I.V. pole, as shown.

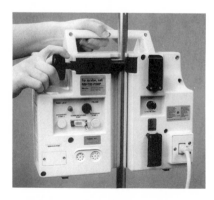

Make sure the display screen is visible and the key board accessible. Plug the cord into a wall outlet.

2 Spike the intravenous container and prime the tubing. Remember to use the standard Baxter solution administration set with the Flo-Gard 6300. After making sure the tubing is primed and all air is expelled from the set, close the set regulating clamp. Now you are ready to insert the I.V. set into the loading mechanism.

3 Raise the pump door latch and pull the door open.

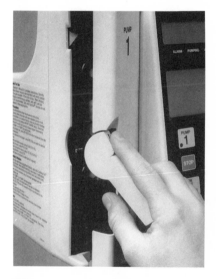

4 Press the safety clamp to the open position.

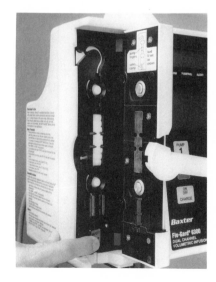

5 Load the I.V. set through the guide channel from top to bottom as shown. Be careful not to misload the I.V. set. Close the pump door.

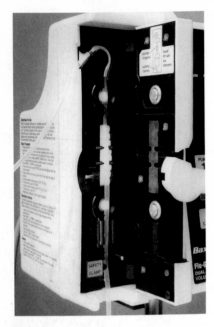

6 Open the set regulating clamp. Check to confirm that no drops of solution are falling in the drip chamber. If you see any flow, close the regulating clamp and recheck I.V. set loading. If you still see flow, do not use this pump.

7 Attach the I.V. set to the venipuncture device. Carefully check the patient's I.V. solution against the doctor's order to verify it is the correct solution before beginning the infusion.

8 Turn the pump on by pressing ON/OFF CHARGE. Verify that the pump performs a self-test. Observe the pump 1 message on the display panel.

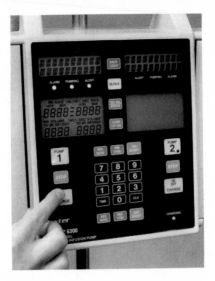

9 Set the volume knob on the rear of the device to the desired alarm tone.

How to program the Flo-gard primary line

The steps to program pump 1 and pump 2 are identical. To select the desired pump, press the key marked either pump 1 or pump 2.

1 Press the key labeled PRI RATE to program the flow rate. Enter the correct rate by pressing the appropriate numbers on the key board.

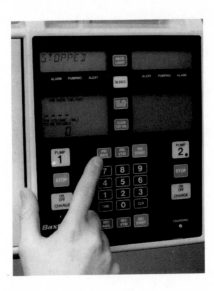

2 Press PRI VTBI to program the primary volume to be infused. Enter the selected volume on the numerical key board.

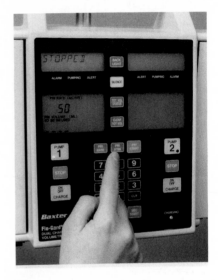

3 If you need to reset the volume previously infused to zero, press CLEAR TOT VOL.

To review infusion settings or to determine total volume infused, press TOT VOL/STATUS. The display will show the volume infused followed by the rate and volume to be infused.

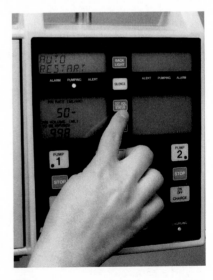

4 To start the infusion, press PRI START. A green pumping light and a moving bar next to the flow rate will indicate the pump is delivering the prescribed solution.

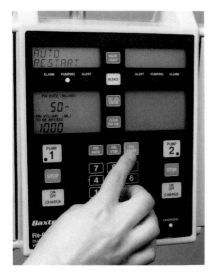

5 If you need to program the other pump, repeat steps 1 through 4.

Learning about the LifeCare 5000 cassette drug delivery system

The LifeCare 5000 Drug Delivery System, commonly called the Plum, combines the features of a pump and a controller. This versatile, cost-efficient infuser can administer a wide range of fluids, drugs, and nutritional products. It allows you to set up a primary line, add a single dose piggyback, and program multidose secondary regimens up to 24 hours in advance. In addition, its variable pressure feature allows you to set a maximum pressure limit. At low pressures, this infuser functions as a controller; at high pressures it functions as a pump.

The Plum, shown above, is a low pressure, dual channel piston-diaphragm pumping system. The Plumset cassette is a component of this system. It permits accurate volumetric delivery and provides safety features such as an air-in-line detec-

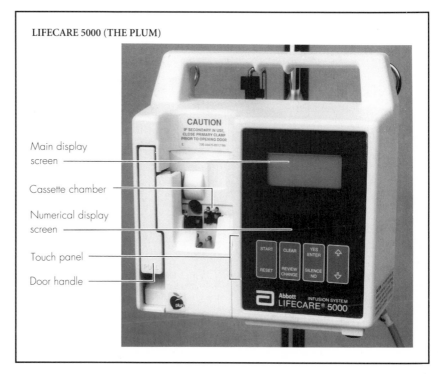

LIFECARE 5000 (THE PLUM)

Main display screen

Cassette chamber

Numerical display screen

Touch panel

Door handle

tor, pressure sensor, and flow regulator. Gravity flow rate is controlled by the cassette flow regulator mechanism, which is similiar in function to the Dial-a-Flow. (You can even use this cassette independently as a flow regulator.) The Plum is small, com-

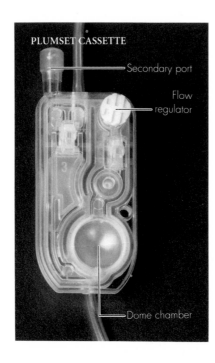

PLUMSET CASSETTE

Secondary port

Flow regulator

Dome chamber

pact, and easy to use. All controls are located on the front panel with prompting messages for infuser operation.

How to set up the Plum primary line

Before using this pump, refer to the manufacturer's manual for instruction on special pump functions.

1 Clamp the pump securely to an I.V. pole.

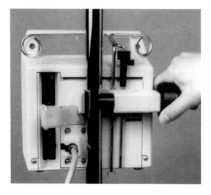

Make sure the display screen is visible and the key board accessible.

Plug the cord into a wall outlet. The Plum will also run on battery power.

2 Remove the Plum cassette from the package. Close the upper slide clamp and the flow regulator.

3 Attach the Plum cassette to the I.V. container and hang the container on the pole. Squeeze and release the drip chamber in the usual manner so it is half full.

4 Open the upper slide clamp. Check to be sure there is no flow in the drip chamber.

5 Invert the cassette inlet tubing so it's facing downward. Open the white plastic flow regulator by turning it counterclockwise. Allow fluid to fill the airtrap (in the next two photographs, the I.V. solution is darkened to show the filling pattern).

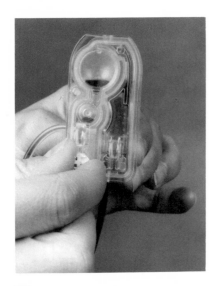

6 When fluid is visible in the upper chamber, turn the cassette back to the upright position as shown. Continue to prime the tubing. Then push in the regulator to close it.

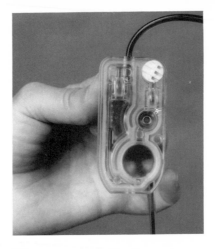

7 Begin the infusion. Open the door latch on the Plum pump and insert the cassette into the guides. Close the door.

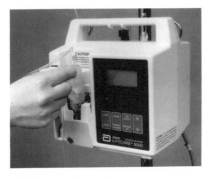

8 The pump will automatically perform a self-test. If the pump checks out, the display screen will read *Self-test OK.*

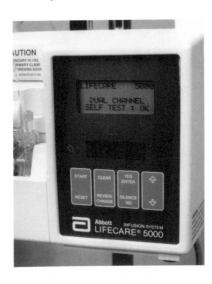

The screen will read *Rate 0 ml/hour.* The first prompt will appear on the screen; it will read: *Press the up or down arrow or Enter.*

9 To set a rate of 50 ml/hour, press the up arrow until this value appears in the display column. Then press ENTER.

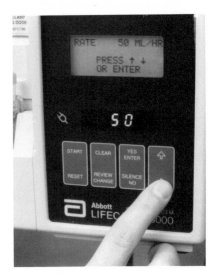

The screen will read *Dose Lim 0 ml.* Now the second prompt will appear on the screen: *Press the up or down arrow or Enter.*

10 To enter a dose of 500 ml, press the up arrow until this value is reached on the screen.

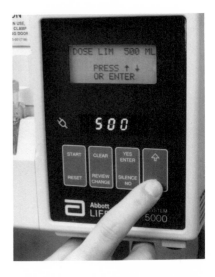

11 Press START to begin the infusion. The display screen will read *Pumping* at the rate you've chosen.

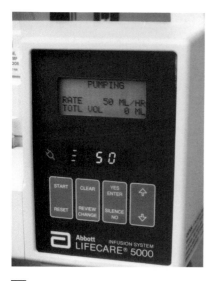

12 A red bar will move up and down to indicate pumping. To review your setting, press REVIEW. The screen will read: *Rate 50 ml/hr, Dose Lim 500 ml, Dose Del 3 ml, Totl Vol 3 ml.* Always review your settings before leaving the patient. Document your actions.

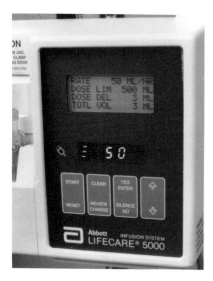

13 This pump also allows you to constantly monitor and read line pressure. For a display of the line pressure, press REVIEW twice.

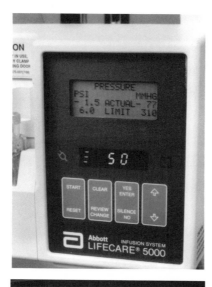

Patient-controlled analgesia pumps

Patient-controlled analgesia (PCA) pumps allow the patient to control I.V. delivery of analgesics (usually morphine) and maintain optimal serum levels. These devices include an infusion pump (joined to a timing unit) and a syringe that delivers a continuous maintenance dosage of an analgesic at a controlled rate. By depressing a button attached to a cord, the patient triggers delivery of a drug dose. The timing unit prevents overdose by imposing a lock-out time (usually 5 to 10 minutes) between doses.

Used for acute or chronic pain, the PCA pump may be especially useful in postoperative and terminal cancer patients. Better pain control may result in fewer postoperative complications and shorter recovery time because immediate drug delivery eases the patient's anxiety and promotes patient compliance with coughing, deep breathing, and ambulation. Compared with intermittent administration, the PCA pump reduces analgesic dosage.

The Travenol Basal-Bolus Infusor (shown on the right), a disposable, nonelectronic, nonbattery PCA and drug administration device, contains an infuser with an accessory patient control module (shown on the left) that's worn like a wristwatch.

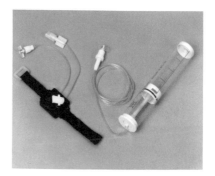

The lightweight, disposable infuser uses an inflatable reservoir (balloon) to deliver the drug at a constant rate. The elastomeric balloon serves as a storage chamber and provides energy for drug infusion. As the balloon deflates, pressure on the fluid produces a prolonged, constant flow. The infuser leads into the watchlike module, which is attached to an I.V. line. The patient requests analgesia by pushing a button on the module, as shown. No more than 0.5 ml of solution can be delivered per lockout period (this device features a 15 minute lock-out period). This infuser combines economical drug control with patient convenience.

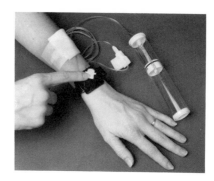

Learning about the Infusaid implantable pump

The Infusaid implantable pump is a palm-sized device powered by a bellows system. Models have one or two sideports, which permit bolus injections, injection of radiopaque dye, and supplemental infusions. A dual-catheter model permits the doctor to treat two different sites or to provide a combination of local and systemic therapy.

During the insertion procedure, the doctor places the pump's catheter in the targeted organ or vessel. He sutures the pump into a subcutaneous pocket created in chest or abdominal tissue (depending on the catheter site). The pump then delivers precise drug doses from its drug reservoir directly to the target area, permitting more effective drug delivery with fewer systemic side effects. For regional chemotherapy, the pump can treat the liver, head, neck, and central nervous system (CNS).

The pump has no external catheters or exit sites, a feature that minimizes the risk of infection. Consequently, it requires no dressing or special care. Because the reservoir can be refilled by injection in the doctor's office, the patient is able to participate in normal activities during therapy.

The Infusaid pump can deliver floxuridine (FUDR), fluorouracil (5-FU), methotrexate, morphine, amikacin (Amikin), heparin, glycerol, saline solution, and bacteriostatic water. Other drugs under study for pump administration include antibiotics for treatment of osteomyelitis, drugs to treat CNS disorders, and additional antineoplastic drugs.

INFUSAID IMPLANTABLE PUMP

This pump's design provides a virtually unlimited power source. When the inner chamber (the drug reservoir) fills with fluid, the bellows expand. The bellows, in turn, compress the outer chamber, which contains a two-phase charging fluid. During drug administration, the patient's body temperature warms the charging fluid, causing it to expand and compress the bellows. The bellows then force the drug through a bacterial membrane filter and preset flow restrictor. Flow rates range from 1 to 6 ml/day, and reservoir capacity ranges from 23 to 50 ml, depending on the pump model.

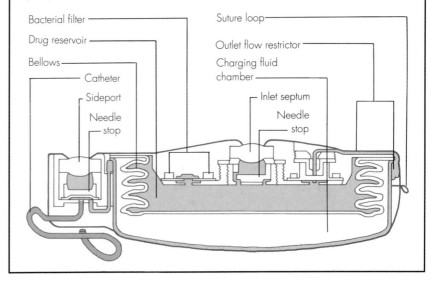

How to refill an Infusaid pump

Besides teaching the patient about his pump, your biggest responsibility may be refilling the pump's drug reservoir. After reviewing the pump's manual, use the following information as a guide.

NOTE Check policy to make sure that refilling an implantable pump is a nursing responsibility in your institution; you may need special certification.

1 Obtain an Infusaid refill kit, which includes a 50-ml syringe barrel (you won't need a plunger), refill tubing with stopcock (0.5-ml capacity), noncoring needles, iodine and alcohol swabsticks, gauze pads, a drape, a pump template, and an adhesive bandage strip. In addition, gather sterile gloves, a 5-ml syringe filled with sterile water for flushing, a 50-ml syringe for drug administration, and the ordered drug. Make sure the drug is warmed to 62° to 95° F (16.7° to 35° C).

NOTE Flushing solutions differ according to catheter site. These examples are given assuming intra-arterial catheter placement.

2 Fill the 50-ml syringe with the warmed drug.

NOTE Only Infusaid pump models 100 and 400 have a 50-ml drug capacity. If you're using another model, consult the manual for instructions.

3 Wash your hands, then gently palpate the pump to find its perimeter.

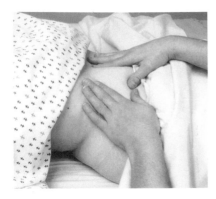

4 Next, find the inlet septum, located near the pump's center and indented about ¼" (0.6 cm). Don't rely on puncture marks from previous refills; the skin may have shifted slightly over the pump.

5 Open the sterile refill kit, put on sterile gloves, prepare the pump site with the alcohol and iodine swabsticks provided in the kit, and drape the area.

6 Attach the 50-ml syringe barrel, as shown, and the noncoring needle

the tubing and stopcock. (An optional luer lock injection site is provided with the tubing set.)

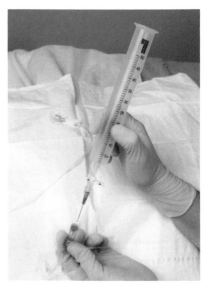

7 To help locate the septum, place the template over the pump, as shown. (If you can palpate the septum easily, you may omit this step.)

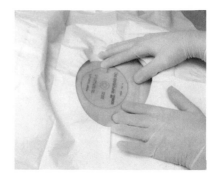

8 Insert the noncoring needle into the septum at a 90-degree angle.

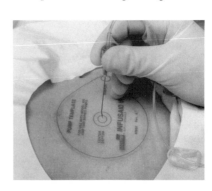

NURSING CONSIDERATIONS: INFUSAID PUMP

To ensure safe, effective drug therapy, keep these special considerations in mind.

Maintaining accurate flow rates
Refill the Infusaid pump with only the drugs or fluids it's designed to deliver. Flow rate is factory set. Refer to the Infusaid pump performance data sheet packaged with the pump for details on dosage and infusion volume.

To ensure dosage accuracy throughout therapy, remember that these factors affect flow rate:
• *atmospheric pressure.* High altitudes, air travel, and reduced atmospheric pressure increase flow rate.
• *body temperature.* Above 98.6° F (37° C), drug flow increases 10% to 13% for each 1-degree rise. A temperature drop reduces flow rate in the same proportions.
• *blood pressure.* Flow rate diminishes 3% for each 10 mm Hg that average arterial blood pressure rises above 90 mm Hg. Flow rate

increases in the same proportions when average arterial blood pressure drops below 90 mm Hg.
• *drug concentration and viscosity.* Some drugs, such as heparin, have concentration-dependent viscosities that affect flow rate. Consult the performance data sheet for guidance.

Patient teaching
Teach your patient how the pump functions and how to avoid problems. For example, tell him to:
• avoid contact sports
• consult his doctor before traveling by plane or to high altitudes
• avoid deep-sea diving and scuba diving
• avoid long, hot baths and saunas
• report fever immediately
• report any unusual symptoms related to drug therapy
• keep all appointments for drug refills
• carry an Infusaid patient-identification card.

9 Open the stopcock and allow the pump to empty. Never aspirate fluid from the pump; aspiration may draw blood into the catheter and cause an occlusion.

10 Note the volume of returned fluid (the syringe barrel has been pre-calibrated to account for tubing volume of 0.5 ml).

If no fluid returns, remove the syringe barrel and replace it with a 5-ml syringe filled with sterile water. Inject the water, release pressure on the plunger, and wait for fluid to return. If necessary, repeat the procedure once. If no fluid returns, stop the procedure and report the problem. Pump failure may be responsible.

11 Close the stopcock; then remove and discard the syringe barrel and stopcock. Leave the needle and tubing in place.

12 Attach the drug-filled syringe to the tubing. Then inject 5 ml of drug into the pump, using both hands as shown.

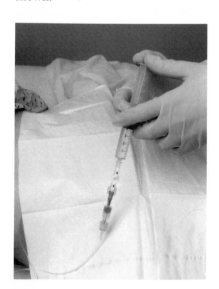

13 Reconfirm needle placement by releasing pressure on the plunger and looking for drug return in the syringe. Then inject the remaining drug in 5-ml increments, rechecking needle placement between increments. After you've injected the ordered dose, maintain pressure on the plunger. Quickly pull out the needle, remove the template, clean iodine from the patient's skin, and apply an adhesive bandage strip.

How to give a bolus dose through an Infusaid sideport

1 Gather the following equipment: an Infusaid refill kit, two 10-ml syringes filled with heparinized normal saline (100 U/ml), a syringe filled with the drug dose, and sterile gloves.

NOTE Use only 10 ml or larger syringes for sideport injection.

2 Wash your hands. Palpate to locate the pump's perimeter, inlet septum, and sideport.

3 Put on gloves, then prepare and drape the site. You may position the template over the pump to help locate the sideport septum.

4 Attach the syringe filled with heparinized saline to the noncoring needle, tubing, and stopcock. Tighten all connections, flush tubing, and close the stopcock.

5 Insert the noncoring needle into the sideport septum at a 90-degree angle.

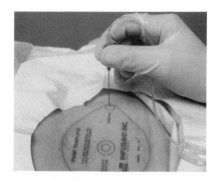

6 Open the stopcock and inject the heparinized saline to flush the catheter. Maintain positive pressure on the syringe plunger. Then close the stopcock as shown and remove and discard the syringe. Examine the puncture site closely for any subcutaneous infiltration.

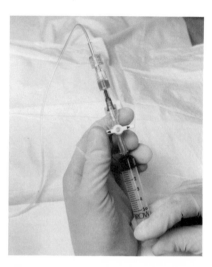

7 Attach the drug-filled syringe to the tubing and open the stopcock. Slowly inject the drug. *Caution:* Limit the injection rate to 10 ml over 1 minute to avoid overpressurizing the sideport.

8 After injecting the drug, maintain positive pressure on the plunger, close the stopcock as shown in step 6, and remove the syringe. Attach the second syringe of heparinized saline to the tubing, open the stopcock, and flush the catheter.

9 Maintaining positive pressure on the plunger, close the stopcock and withdraw the needle from the sideport. Remove the template, clean iodine from the patient's skin, if necessary, and apply the adhesive bandage strip.

Learning about subcutaneous access devices

Designed primarily for patients who need prolonged or intermittent I.V. treatment, a subcutaneous access device provides I.V. access for bolus or continuous infusion without repeated venipuncture. Because all the components lie under the skin, the device doesn't need a dressing and won't interfere with the patient's body image or normal activities.

The Hickman subcutaneous port shown below is a small disk about

To help prevent clot formation and catheter blockage, the subcutaneous port should be heparinized after each use. When not in use, it should be heparinized according to the manufacturer's instructions and institution policy. Ports are contraindicated whenever:
- infection, bacteremia, or septicemia is known or suspected.
- the patient's body is too small to accommodate the implanted port or catheter.
- the patient is known or suspected

PERIPHERAL PLACEMENT OF A SUBCUTANEOUS PORT

When placement in the patient's chest is contraindicated by intensive surgery and scarring, radiation requirements, disease complications or the patient's fear of additional surgery, a venous access system may be implanted from a peripheral location on the arm.

For such use, a small port (7.4 mm x 26.7 mm) is designed to fit the contour of the arm. Normally, this port is placed in the anterior or lateral upper forearm. The catheter of this system reaches the central venous circulation via the basilic or cephalic vein.

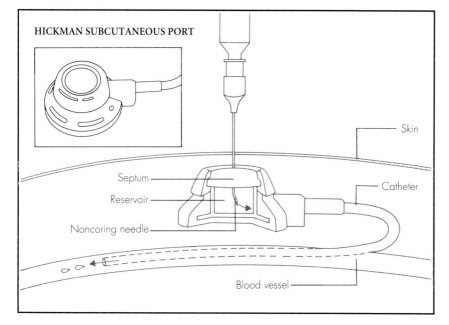

HICKMAN SUBCUTANEOUS PORT

Skin

Septum

Catheter

Reservoir

Noncoring needle

Blood vessel

1½" (3.8 cm) diameter. The port has a raised center or septum over the medication reservoir, which is made of self-sealing rubber material that will sustain up to 2,000 punctures. The catheter is radiopaque silicone rubber, may be preconnected or attached to the port, and is available for intravenous, intra-arterial or peritoneal use (attachable version only). After implantation, the port is visible merely as a small raised area beneath the skin.

to be allergic to materials contained in the device, or hasn't tolerated other implanted devices.

Implantation of the subcutaneous port

Implantation of the port can be performed under local anesthetic and usually takes an hour or less; it is often performed on an outpatient basis.

For maximum stability, the port should lie over a bony structure. It is typically placed in a subcutaneous pocket in the right upper chest. The

catheter is then threaded through the subclavian vein and terminates at the junction of the superior vena cava and the right atrium (see page 154). The doctor sutures the port to the underlying fascia, flushes it with heparin, closes the incision, and confirms placement with an X-ray.

Placement of an intra-arterial port (an inpatient procedure) can locate the port over the ribs with the catheter inserted into the hepatic arterial system. The port with a special attachable peritoneal catheter may be placed over the ribs, with the catheter tunneled to the peritoneal cavity, which allows repeated infusion and withdrawal of drugs or fluids. However, the placement site may vary depending on the patient and clinical considerations.

Postoperative care after placement of a subcutaneous port includes routine inspection of the site for signs of swelling, infection, hematoma, seroma, and erosion, and rotation of the device. Wound care includes cleaning and dressing according to institution protocol.

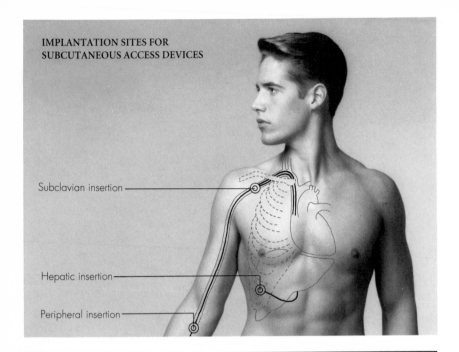

IMPLANTATION SITES FOR
SUBCUTANEOUS ACCESS DEVICES

Subclavian insertion

Hepatic insertion

Peripheral insertion

NURSING CONSIDERATIONS: SUBCUTANEOUS PORT ACCESS

• When administering a continuous infusion, use a right-angled non-coring needle and an extension set. After insertion, the design of this needle will allow the upper portion to lie just above the skin surface and allow easy application of a transparent dressing over the injection site, as shown.

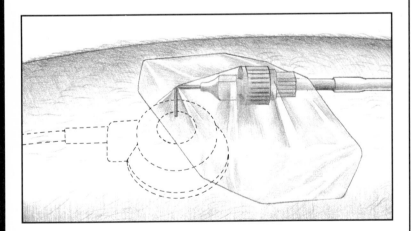

• While policy varies by institution, one manufacturer recommends that unused ports be heparinized as follows: intra-arterial ports, once a week; intravenous ports, once every 4 weeks.

• Flushing with fibrolytic agents has cleared clotted catheters after irrigation, aspiration, and change of body position have failed, but may be used only if the patient's doctor orders it.

How to access the subcutaneous port

Port access is performed by percutaneous needle insertion with a noncoring needle (see *Selecting needles*, page 61).

1 Gather the following equipment: sterile gloves, antiseptic swabs, alcohol swabs, a 22G noncoring needle, a syringe (with needle) containing 5 ml sterile heparinized saline, a 10-ml syringe (with needle) containing sterile normal saline, a 5-ml syringe for blood aspiration, I.V. extension tubing with a clamp, and medication.

Wash your hands. Explain the procedure and warn the patient to expect a needle prick. Administer a topical anesthetic, if ordered.

2 Palpate to locate the reservoir and injection port.

3 Put on gloves and prepare the injection site using a spiral motion over an area 4" to 5" (10 to 13 cm) in diameter, starting at the port and working outward.

4 Flush the extension tubing with sterile normal saline to expel the air. Clamp the tubing and set it and the saline-filled syringe aside.

5 Triangulate the port between the thumb and first two fingers of your nondominant hand as shown.

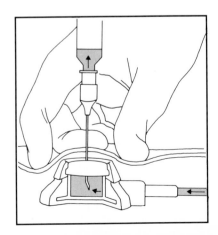

TROUBLESHOOTING PROBLEMS WITH A SUBCUTANEOUS ACCESS DEVICE

PROBLEM	POSSIBLE CAUSE	INTERVENTION
Erythema	Infected incision or port pocket, poor healing postoperatively	Assess daily for redness and drainage. Notify doctor. Administer antibiotics as ordered.
Inability to flush or withdraw from system	Kinked I.V. tubing	Check tubing.
	Pump malfunction	Check equipment.
	Catheter lodged against the vein wall	Reposition patient by moving upper torso and arms.
	Incorrect needle placement	Reposition needle and advance tip to the bottom of the reservoir. Verify correct positioning by blood aspiration.
	Fibrin sheath formation	Flush with 3 ml of sterile normal saline and repeat if necessary. Increase frequency of flushing to prevent sheath formation.
	Occlusion (clots)	Use a fibrinolytic agent such as urokinase (Abbokinase), as ordered.
	Kinked catheter, port rotation	Contact doctor.
Burning sensation in subcutaneous tissue	Dislodgement of needle into subcutaneous tissue	Do not remove needle. Stop infusion and immediately notify doctor.

Insert the needle with a dartlike motion at a 90-degree angle over the septum until you feel the needle reach the bottom of the reservoir. Then, attach a 5-ml syringe to the needle hub and aspirate blood to verify needle placement. If you do not confirm placement, do not proceed. Notify the doctor and await further orders.

6 Attach the extension tubing and the saline-filled syringe to the noncoring needle and flush the port with 5 ml of solution. Clamp the extension set and remove the syringe. (If you can't inject the solution, the noncoring needle tip may be positioned incorrectly. Make sure you've advanced it to the needle stop and try to inject the solution. If you still can't inject the solution, remove the needle and start over.) When the injection is complete, clamp the extension set.

7 Connect the syringe containing the drug to the extension set. Release the clamp and administer the bolus injection. When the injection is complete, clamp the extension set.

Remember to examine the injection site for signs of extravasation; if noted, immediately discontinue the injection and notify the doctor.

8 Flush the extension tubing with 5 ml sterile saline solution and then with 5 ml sterile heparinized saline to prevent clot formation and catheter blockage.

9 To remove the noncoring needle, stabilize the reservoir between your thumb and forefinger. Then withdraw the needle, taking care not to twist or angle it. After needle withdrawal, you may see a slight amount of serosanguineous discharge at the puncture site.

Insulin infusion pumps

By delivering basal (small) insulin doses every few minutes and bolus doses at mealtimes, an insulin infusion pump helps a diabetic patient exert better control over blood glucose levels and minimizes long-term complications.

The MiniMed pump

The MiniMed insulin pump shown here is about the size of a deck of cards and resembles a beeper.

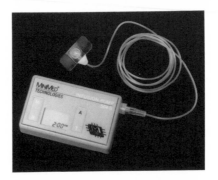

Its case holds three disposable batteries to power the pump. The syringe inside holds regular insulin. A tiny computer inside the pump controls the action of the syringe and precisely regulates how much insulin the pump delivers. The pump can deliver up to four different basal rates in a 24-hour period. These rates and their associated delivery times are called *profiles.* Insulin is delivered through an infusion set and exits through a needle inserted under the skin.

UNDERSTANDING MINIMED BUTTONS

The MiniMed pump has four buttons and a display screen. These buttons are used to program the pump, while the screen displays messages.

M button: Meal bolus, used to set the amount of insulin given before a meal.

B button: Basal rate, used to set the amount of insulin delivered every hour during a 24-hour period.

A button: Activates the pump to carry out selected program.

T button: Time of day, used to set the time of day.

HOW TO CALCULATE INSULIN PUMP DOSAGE

BASAL GUIDELINE
Basal dosage = 50% of prepump total

Average basal rate requirements
Most patients require doses that fall within the range of 0.4 to 2 U/hour. The average basal rate requirement is 0.7 to 0.9 U/hour.

BOLUS ALGORITHMS
Bolus algorithms reflect a method of adjusting insulin dosages based on guidelines set by the clinician. For instance, if a patient usually takes a 5-U bolus before lunch and has a blood glucose of 275 mg/dl before lunch, the algorithm you provide might instruct the patient to take an 8-U bolus.

Guidelines for determining bolus algorithms
• On average, 1 U of insulin lowers the blood glucose level 40 mg/dl, but it varies from 20 to 80 mg/dl. Most doctors use 1 U per 50 mg/dl as a safe starting point.
• The amount that 1 U of insulin will lower the blood glucose level depends on many factors and should be adjusted for each patient.
• Because insulin sensitivity varies, experimentation is necessary to

determine the exact dosage for each patient. To determine this dosage, patients should keep careful diaries that record boluses and resultant blood glucoses values. Reviewing these results can determine the effect of 1 U of insulin on the blood glucose level.

TIMING OF BOLUS DOSES
Bolus calculations should be modified with individual algorithms for each patient. To determine the correct schedule and dose of a bolus before a meal, patients should:
• check blood glucose level 30 to 45 minutes before a meal.
• use the algorithm to determine the bolus dose.
  If the blood glucose level is in the desired range, the patient can administer the bolus and eat 30 minutes later.
  If the blood glucose level is hyperglycemic (greater than150 mg/dl), the patient should administer the bolus but wait approximately 1 hour before eating. Patient should check blood glucose again and eat when blood glucose is less than150 mg/dl.
  If the blood glucose level is hypoglycemic (less than 80 mg/dl), the patient should administer the bolus and eat immediately. If food is unavailable, the patient should not administer the bolus.

Waterproof tape holds the needle in place. The patient can also choose the nonneedle (Sof-set) system in which a tiny plastic tube with a needle is inserted into the skin. The needle is then removed, leaving only the tube in place. The Sof-set can be placed in the abdomen, thigh, or flank, and should be changed every 2 to 3 days.

Advantages over conventional insulin injection

Small, frequent insulin doses released automatically, with extra doses at mealtimes, permit better blood glucose control, thus reducing long-term diabetic complications. Because the patient can adjust insulin dosage as needed, he can be more flexible about what and when he eats.

The best candidates for insulin pump therapy include:
• patients whose blood glucose levels fluctuate widely despite optimal insulin and dietary regimens
• patients with variable work schedules or mealtimes
• pregnant women, who may have a healthier pregnancy with more precise blood glucose control

DOCUMENTATION

To document use of the MiniMed insulin pump, press the buttons listed below to retrieve the desired information.

• Basal rate	B
• Meal bolus	M
• Total insulin	M/B
• Profiles (if any)	
1st profile	B/T
2nd profile	B/T/T
3rd profile	B/T/T/T
4th profile	B/T/T/T/T

CLASSIFYING GLUCOSE-INTOLERANCE DISORDERS

The National Diabetes Data Group of the National Institutes of Health recognizes these categories of diabetes mellitus and other related conditions.

CATEGORY	FORMER TERMS
Diabetes mellitus	
Type I: Insulin-dependent diabetes mellitus (IDDM)	• Juvenile diabetes, juvenile-onset diabetes, ketosis-prone diabetes, unstable or brittle diabetes
Type II: Non-insulin-dependent diabetes mellitus (NIDDM) • Nonobese NIDDM • Obese NIDDM (includes families with autosomal dominant inheritance)	• Adult-onset diabetes, maturity-onset diabetes, acidosis-resistant diabetes, stable diabetes
Other types, including diabetes mellitus associated with pancreatic disease; hormonal, drug- or chemical-induced disorders; certain genetic syndromes; insulin receptor abnormalities	• Secondary diabetes
Impaired glucose tolerance (IGT)	
Nonobese IGT Obese IGT	• Asymptomatic diabetes, chemical diabetes, latent diabetes, borderline diabetes, subclinical diabetes
IGT associated with pancreatic disease; hormonal, drug- or chemical-induced disorders; insulin receptor abnormalities; certain genetic syndromes	
Gestational diabetes	
Occurs only during pregnancy	• Gestational diabetes
Statistical risk classes	
Previous abnormality: patients now have normal tolerance but previously had diabetic hyperglycemia or IGT, either spontaneously or in response to a known stimulus; includes former gestational and obese diabetics and others with transient hyperglycemia	• Subclinical diabetes, prediabetes, latent diabetes
Potential abnormality: includes persons who have never had abnormal glucose tolerance but who are at increased risk for diabetes because of age, weight, race, or family history	• Prediabetes, potential diabetes

• children or teenagers who aren't developing normally or who experience blood glucose fluctuations related to puberty.

Patient requirements

Insulin pump therapy requires that the patient know the basics of insulin pharmacology and blood glucose self-monitoring. He must also adhere to appropriate diet and exercise regimens. Consequently, the doctor probably won't order insulin pump therapy for patients who:
• won't or can't comply with standard dietary, insulin, and self-monitoring regimens.
• miss medical appointments.
• can't recognize hypoglycemia.

Patients with severe diabetic complications, such as advanced renal disease, proliferative retinopathy, or severe autonomic neuropathy, may also be poor candidates.

Continous subcutaneous infusions for pain control

When oral opioid administration is not feasible because an extremely high dosage is required or because the patient has nausea, dysphagia, or breathing difficulty, continuous subcutaneous infusion (CSI) is an excellent alternative.

CSI is performed with a 25G to 27G subcutaneous needle inserted at a 30- to 45-degree angle; a portable infusion pump is necessary for accurate delivery. Appropriate insertion sites include the supraclavicular area, anterior chest wall, abdomen, and thighs. Sites should be rotated every 2 to 7 days. After insertion, the site is covered with a transparent dressing.

CSI is economical, allows increased patient mobility, decreases patient apprehension, and permits easier patient teaching. However, CSI has a limited infusion volume, prolongs achievement of peak serum opioid levels, and carries the risk of fibrous plaque formation and subsequent irregular absorption and perfusion.

When selecting patients who might benefit from CSI for pain control, consider the following factors:
• available subcutaneous tissue. Attempting CSI in a patient without adequate subcutaneous tissue causes poor absorption and perfusion and, as a result, inadequate pain control.
• required opioid dosage and necessary delivery fluid volume. Subcutaneous tissue can't absorb more than 1 to 2 ml/hour.

The Kangaroo feeding pump

Electronic infusion pumps are used to administer continuous enteral feedings, which occasionally include the addition of medication (see How to Give Medication Through a Gastrostomy Tube, pages 23 and 24). If the doctor wants a patient to receive continuous feedings, consider using a volumetric pump. A pump is more dependable than a gravity administration set because of its constant flow rate and built in safety features.

KANGAROO FEEDING PUMP

Designed to regulate the flow rate of enteral feedings, the Sherwood Medical Kangaroo feeding pump is a rotary peristaltic pump that runs from a wall outlet or battery power. A fully charged battery will operate the pump for up to 24 hours at a rate of 125 ml/hour. Small and lightweight, this device requires the use of a Kangaroo pump set; it will not operate with other feeding sets. This pump offers touch panel operation for easy programming and built in safety features. The pump triggers an audible and visible alarm when it fails to maintain programmed delivery. Before using this pump, refer to the manufacturer's operating manual.

A Handle

B Upper drip chamber guide (including drop sensor)

C Tubing guide

D Lower drip chamber guide

E Retainer lock

F Rotor assembly

G Touch panel

H LED display and pump running indicator lights

I Power cord connector

J Alarm volume control knob

K AC light

L Vol CLR light

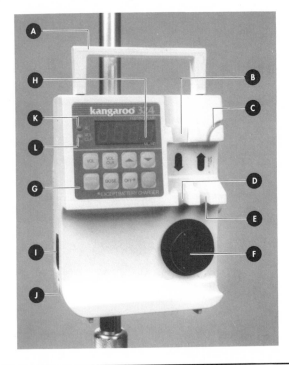

Parenteral Nutrition

When to administer parenteral nutrition

Parenteral nutrition involves the administration of a solution containing dextrose, proteins, electrolytes, vitamins, trace elements, and fat emulsions through a central catheter or a peripheral vein. Parenteral nutrition is prescribed for patients who can't get adequate nutrition with a standard diet or through oral or enteral feeding. It may be indicated for patients with:
• anorexia nervosa
• bowel fistulas
• bowel obstruction
• burns
• Crohn's disease
• gastric carcinoma
• malabsorption syndrome
• multisystem trauma
• obstructive esophageal carcinoma
• pancreatitis
• peritonitis
• regional enteritis
• short-bowel syndrome
• ulcerative colitis.

It is not indicated in patients who:
• are terminally ill and have had all therapy discontinued.
• have bleeding abnormalities or hypercoagulation.
• have an obstructed or partially thrombosed superior vena cava with central line administration.

Standard hypertonic solutions used in parenteral nutrition must be administered through a central line. You will be able to administer only a specially prepared isotonic or slightly hypertonic nutritional solution through a peripheral vein. A specially prepared nutritional solution is also required for patients with renal or hepatic failure (see *Basic formulas for total parenteral nutrition*).

Understanding common additives

Common components of parenteral nutrition solutions include dextrose 50% in water, amino acids, and any number of additives, prescribed to treat a patient's metabolic deficiencies, including those listed here.
• **Potassium:** needed for cellular activity and tissue synthesis
• **Folic acid:** necessary for DNA synthesis; promotes growth and development
• **Vitamin D:** essential for bone metabolism and maintenance of serum calcium levels
• **Trace minerals:** (MTE-5 contains zinc, manganese, chromium, copper, selenium) help wounds heal, aid metabolism of nutrients, act as catalysts in enzyme systems, prevent specific deficiencies
• **Sodium:** helps control water distribution and maintain normal fluid balance
• **Chloride:** regulates the acid-base balance and maintains osmotic pressure
• **Vitamin B complex:** helps in final absorption of carbohydrates and protein

---

BASIC FORMULAS FOR TOTAL PARENTERAL NUTRITION

The feeding formula for total parenteral nutrition (TPN) is prepared according to the patient's needs as ordered by the doctor. The formulas listed below are commonly used.

FORMULA	DEXTROSE	AMINO ACIDS
Standard formula Supplies: 8 g nitrogen, 850 carbohydrate calories, 1,050 total calories	50% (500 ml)	10% (500 ml)
Low carbohydrate formula Supplies: 8 g nitrogen, 510 carbohydrate calories, 710 total calories	30% (500 ml)	10% (500 ml)
Hepatic failure formula Supplies: 6 g nitrogen, 850 carbohydrate calories, 1,010 total calories	50% (500 ml)	8% (500 ml)
Peripheral formula Supplies: 6 g nitrogen, 170 carbohydrate calories, 310 total calories	10% (500 ml)	7% (500 ml)

• **Calcium:** needed for bone and teeth development; aids in blood clotting
• **Phosphate:** minimizes the threat of peripheral parestheses
• **Magnesium:** helps absorb carbohydrates and protein
• **Acetate:** prevents metabolic acidosis
• **Vitamin K:** helps prevent bleeding disorders
• **Vitamin C:** helps in wound healing
    When using additives, keep these points in mind:
• If the patient is dehydrated from a draining fistula, increased urinary output, or diaphoresis, he will require increased sodium in his daily parenteral nutrition allotment.
• Unless calcium is added to parenteral nutrition solutions that contain phosphate, the patient may develop tetany from a drop in his serum calcium level.

Assembling parenteral nutrition equipment

One of your responsibilities in administering parenteral nutrition therapy is assembling the equipment before insertion of the central line. Prepackaged central venous catheterization kits containing the necessary equipment are available. Assemble the following supplies and make sure everything is in working order:
• cassette tubing with 0.22-micron filter (1.2 micron filter if fat emulsion is added to the solution)
• dextrose 5% in water
• infusion pump
• intravenous tubing
• parenteral nutrition solution.

NOTE Sterile conditions are particularly crucial in parenteral nutrition therapy. Observe strict aseptic technique whenever you're handling the equipment.

Learning about 3-in-1 total parenteral nutrition solutions

Three-in-one total parenteral nutrition (TPN) admixtures combine dextrose, amino acids, fat emulsions, electrolytes, trace elements, and vitamins all in the same container. They contain a mixture of 2 or 3 liters in a 3 liter bag; the mixture is administered peripherally or centrally over 24 hours.
    Three-in-one TPN solutions offer:
• cost savings through reduction in labor and supplies
• time savings for the nurse (or patient) because container is added only once in 24 hours.
• convenience for home treatment because it doesn't require frequent interruption of patient's activities.
    Disadvantages include:
• opacity of the emulsion prevents a visual check for particles in the container.
• risk of fat embolism from an unstable emulsion.
• loss of a 24-hour supply of feeding solution if the patient needs a formula change.
    When administering 3-in-1 TPN solutions:
• follow institution policy for administering such solutions.
• ensure that admixtures are compatible.
• discard the solution if you notice cracking of the fat emulsion (layering or oily bubbles in the solution).
• use a 1.2-micron filter.
• administer with an infusion pump.
• observe for complications.

Administering I.V. fat emulsions

You'll probably give I.V. fat emulsions to a patient who:
• needs calories and can't tolerate the high percentage of dextrose in parenteral nutrition solutions.
• needs protein and nitrogen supplements, such as a patient with cancer, stenosis, or a peptic ulcer.

NURSING CONSIDERATIONS: TPN

• Observe strict aseptic technique. Infection is a serious threat because of the solution's high sugar content and the patient's weakened state. *Candida, Staphylococcus aureus, S. epidermidis,* or *Klebsiella* infection is likely.
• Never take a blood sample or a central venous pressure reading, use a three-way stopcock, or piggyback a solution on a TPN line.
• Always infuse the solution at a constant rate with an infusion pump. To avoid complications such as hyperglycemia, hyperosmolarity, or fluid overload, don't interrupt treatment, don't infuse the solution too rapidly, and never try to catch up on feedings that are behind schedule.
• If any of the equipment becomes contaminated, or the catheter develops a leak, change the entire I.V. setup.
• Watch for and promptly report signs of infection: redness, swelling, oozing, pus, or fever.
• Watch for signs of thrombosis. Call the doctor if the patient has pain or soreness in his chest, shoulder, or neck; swelling in his catheterized arm; or neck vein distention.
• Watch for infiltration from catheter rupture or vessel erosion: swelling in the chest, neck, and shoulder area and burning or hardening of tissues. If in doubt, stop the infusion. A chest X-ray should be taken.

DEALING WITH COMPLICATIONS OF T.P.N.

If your patient is receiving TPN, you need to be aware of potential complications. Major complications of TPN therapy may be catheter related, metabolic, or mechanical.

POSSIBLE COMPLICATIONS	WHAT TO WATCH FOR	TREATMENT
Catheter related		
Pneumothorax and hydrothorax	Dyspnea, chest pain, cyanosis, decreased breath sounds	Suction; insert chest tube.
Brachial plexus injury	Tingling and numbness along arm in peripheral TPN catheters	Remove catheter.
Air embolism	Apprehension, chest pain, tachycardia, hypotension, cyanosis, seizure, loss of consciousness, cardiopulmonary arrest	Clamp catheter. Place patient in the Trendelenburg position on left side. Give oxygen as ordered. If cardiac arrest occurs, perform CPR with patient on his left side. Keep patient in this position until asymptomatic.
Sepsis	Fever, chills, leukocytosis, erythema or pus at insertion site	Remove catheter and remove tip for culture. Start appropriate antibiotics.
Metabolic		
Hyperglycemia	Polyuria, dehydration, elevated blood and urine glucose levels	Start insulin therapy or adjust flow rate.
Hyperosmolar nonketotic syndrome	Confusion, lethargy, seizures, coma, hyperglycemia, dehydration, glycosuria	Stop dextrose. Give insulin and 0.45% NaCl to rehydrate.
Hypokalemia	Muscle weakness, paralysis, paresthesias, arrhythmias	Increase potassium supplementation.
Hypomagnesemia	Tingling around mouth, paresthesias in fingers, mental changes, hyperreflexia	Increase magnesium supplementation.
Hypophosphatemia	Irritability, weakness, paresthesias, coma, respiratory arrest	Increase phosphate supplementation.
Hypocalcemia	Paresthesias, twitching, positive Chvostek's sign, decreased serum bicarbonate level	Increase calcium supplementation.
Metabolic acidosis	Increased serum chloride level, decreased serum bicarbonate level	Use acetate or lactate salts of Na^+ or H^+.
Hepatic dysfunction	Increased serum transaminases, lactic dehydrogenase, and bilirubin levels	Use special hepatic formulations. Decrease carbohydrate, and add I.V. fats.

continued

DEALING WITH COMPLICATIONS OF T.P.N. *continued*

POSSIBLE COMPLICATIONS	WHAT TO WATCH FOR	TREATMENT
Metabolic *continued*		
Hypoglycemia	Sweating, shaking, irritability when infusion is stopped	Infuse with dextrose 10% in water.
Mechanical		
Obstruction of catheter lumen	Interrupted flow rate, hypoglycemia	Reposition catheter. Attempt to aspirate clot. If unsuccessful, instill urokinase (Abbokinase) as a fibrinolytic agent to clear catheter.
Air embolism	Apprehension, chest pain, tachycardia, hypotension, cyanosis, seizure, loss of consciousness, cardiopulmonary arrest	Clamp catheter. Place patient in the Trendelenburg position on left side. Give oxygen as ordered. If cardiac arrest occurs, perform CPR with patient on his left side. Keep patient in this position until asymptomatic.
Thrombosis	Erythema and edema at puncture site; ipsilateral swelling of arm, neck, or face; pain along vein; malaise; fever, tachycardia	Remove catheter promptly. Administer anticoagulant doses of heparin, if ordered. Venous flow studies may be done.
Fluid extravasation	Swelling of neck and shoulder area on affected side, pain	Stop I.V. infusion. Observe patient for cardiopulmonary abnormalities by assessment and chest X-ray.

• needs more essential fatty acids than are contained in TPN solutions.
• needs nutritional improvement, for example, before surgery.

Don't give an I.V. fat emulsion to the patient who has:
• a disturbance of normal fat metabolism, such as hyperlipemia.
• severe hepatic disease. (Remember, the liver helps utilize fatty acids.)
• a blood coagulation defect caused by a decreased blood platelet count.
• a pulmonary disease.
• lipoid nephrosis.
• hepatocellular damage.
• bone marrow dyscrasia.
• received treatment with anabolic inhibitory drugs.

Notify the doctor if the patient develops any of the following reactions.

Within 2½ hours:
• fever
• flushing
• sweating
• pressure sensations over eyes
• nausea
• vomiting
• headache
• chest and back pains
• dyspnea, cyanosis.

Within 10 days:
• hepatomegaly
• splenomegaly
• thrombocytopenia
• focal seizures
• hyperlipemia
• hepatic damage, jaundice
• hemorrhagic diathesis
• gastroduodenal ulcer.

NURSING CONSIDERATIONS: I.V. FAT EMULSIONS

• Use an electronic control device to maintain an even flow rate and avoid fatty-acid overload. Regularly measure the patient's fluid intake and output, caloric intake, and temperature. Take daily blood samples to determine the triglyceride level. Document your findings.
• If the patient's receiving long-term treatment with an I.V. fat emulsion, monitor his ability to eliminate the infused fat. Perform hepatic function tests; if function's impaired, inform the doctor.

Blood Transfusions

Learning about blood transfusions

You may see blood being transfused every day and think it's a simple matter. But don't be misled. Blood transfusion's a very complex procedure. Whether the patient's health benefits from the transfusion depends largely on your knowledge and ability. You should know:
• the differences among administration sets
• how to use special accessory equipment
• why the doctor may choose a blood component rather than whole blood
• how to reduce the risk of transmitting human immunodeficiency virus
• what complications may arise from a transfusion, and how to treat them.

If you're not familiar with these specifics, read the following pages carefully.

What blood does

Blood plays a fundamental role in maintaining the body. It carries everything the tissues require for energy or synthesis, and removes all cellular waste products. Blood:
• supplies oxygen and nutrients for tissue maintenance, growth, and repair
• transports cellular waste, including carbon dioxide, to the elimination organs
• provides a defense against infection by transporting antibodies
• regulates and equalizes body temperature
• helps to maintain the tissues' acid-base balance
• regulates the tissues' water and electrolyte content.

Guidelines for transfusing blood components

Whenever you administer blood components, take great care to avoid mistakes. Proper identification and matching procedures are crucial. Also be sure to consider use of filters and blood warmers, needle size, and administration rate. Stay alert, too, for potential complications. Before transfusing blood components, follow these guidelines to prevent transfusion hazards.

Ask the patient who has had a blood transfusion before how he felt during and after the procedure. Report any history of adverse reaction during or after a previous blood transfusion to the doctor and the hospital blood bank. A patient who's had repeated febrile, nonhemolytic transfusion reactions may benefit from leukocyte-poor blood components.

If the patient has never had a blood transfusion, explain the procedure and tell the patient why the transfusion has been ordered. Above all, tell him to report any symptoms of an adverse reaction, such as headache or chills.

Finally, make sure the patient signs a consent form, if required, before he receives the transfusion.

Use a 16G, 18G, or 20G needle or cannula to administer whole blood or packed red blood cells (RBCs). If vein access is poor, you may infuse blood using a 22G or 24G cannula, but you may need a blood pump to ensure an adequate rate. A 21G or 23G winged administration set can be used for small veins and in infants. However, small-gauge plastic cannulas are preferred; they have a lower risk of infiltration. When pumps

aren't used, you may dilute packed cells with normal saline solution and increase head pressure by raising the I.V. pole to aid blood flow when using smaller-gauge needles.

Determine filter use

Ordinarily, a 170-micron blood filter is used for blood transfusions. Albumin, however, comes packaged with its own filter tubing. Blood tubing has a large screen filter, which removes fibrin clots and other debris. Microaggregate filters of 20 to 40 microns are used for patients with pulmonary impairment, although some hospitals use them routinely for multiple transfusions. These filters remove white blood cells (WBCs) and smaller microaggregates. They're used only for whole blood or packed RBCs, never for plasma or platelets (they screen out platelets). If used to remove WBCs from packed cells, microaggregate filters eliminate the need to wash RBCs. These filters produce a slower flow rate than a standard filter.

To evaluate the patient's response to a blood transfusion accurately, you must take baseline vital signs before the transfusion. Clinicians also recommend taking vital signs several times during the first 15 minutes after you start the transfusion.

Remember, however, that careful observation of the patient during and after a blood transfusion will provide a more reliable assessment of his condition than just taking vital signs. The patient may be more likely to complain of discomfort, or to show some sign of an adverse reaction, before his vital signs change. (See *Transfusion risks: Immediate reactions,* pages 174 and 175.)

(Text continues on page 168.)

GUIDE TO BLOOD PRODUCTS

Because blood has so many important functions, any deficiency requires correction. The chart below outlines which blood products are needed to correct specific deficiencies.

BLOOD PRODUCT	DESCRIPTION	INDICATIONS	EQUIPMENT
Whole blood	500-ml unit contains about 200 ml of red blood cells (RBCs) and 300 ml of plasma	• Massive blood loss • Exchange transfusion in neonates	• Large-gauge needle or catheter (18G or 19G for adults, 22G or 23G for neonates, children, and adults with small veins) • Normal saline for starter solution • Blood administration set containing in-line blood filter with 170-micron pore size and standard size surface area • Multiple-lead tubing (preferably a Y set) recommended; straight tubing may be used but isn't recommended
Red blood cells (packed)	350- to 400-ml unit contains about 200 to 250 ml of RBCs (with same amount of hemoglobin as whole blood) and 150 ml of plasma and additive solution (saline, adenine, glucose, and mannitol)	• Inadequate oxygen-carrying capacity	• Same as for whole blood, but filter with larger surface area may be used to increase transfusion rate
Red blood cells (deglycerolized or leukocyte poor)	200-ml unit contains RBCs suspended in 50 ml of normal saline, with virtually all leukocytes and plasma proteins removed. Deglycerolized RBCs, taken from donors with rare blood types, are first frozen (with glycerol added to preserve RBCs), then thawed and deglycerolized before transfusion. Leukocyte-poor RBCs aren't frozen.	• Rare blood types (deglycerolized only) • History of repeated febrile non-hemolytic reactions not responsive to other leukocyte depletion methods (leukocyte-poor RBCs only) • Immunoglobulin A (IgA) deficiency with sensitivity to IgA (leukocyte-poor RBCs preferred, but deglycerolized RBCs may be administered)	• Same as for whole blood
Plasma (fresh frozen or single-donor frozen)	200- to 250-ml unit of fresh-frozen plasma and single-donor frozen plasma contain all coagulation factors, plus 250 mg of fibrinogen. (*Single-donor frozen* implies that *fresh-frozen* plasma is pooled from multiple donors; it's not. Term is commonly used, nevertheless.)	• Coagulation deficiencies for which specific factor concentrates are unavailable	• Same as for whole blood, except: –component administration set may be indicated because its filter has smaller surface area that's less likely to trap plasma. –smaller needle or catheter size (22G or 23G for adults) may be used because product is not viscous.

ADMINISTRATION	SPECIAL CONSIDERATIONS
• Obtain blood product within 30 minutes of expected time of transfusion. • Identify blood product and patient (at least two persons must do this). • Take baseline vital signs. • Start transfusion *slowly*. No more than 30 ml should be transfused during first 15 minutes. Stay with patient during this time and watch for adverse reactions. If none occur, establish and maintain prescribed transfusion rate. Entire unit should be transfused in 2 to 4 hours. • Take vital signs frequently throughout transfusion.	• Always administer ABO group- and Rh type-specific
• Same as for whole blood.	• Always administer ABO group- and Rh type-specific. If not, group- and type-compatible can be transfused safely.
• Same as for whole blood.	• Administer ABO group- and Rh type-specific if possible. If not, group- and type-compatible can be transfused safely. • Because of thawing, cells are transferred into container other than original blood bag (such as transfer pack). Unit has 24-hour expiration date from time of thawing or washing. • Risk of febrile nonhemolytic reactions is decreased because virtually all leukocytes are removed. • Risk of anaphylactic and allergic urticarial reactions is decreased because virtually all plasma has been removed.
• Same as for whole blood, but transfuse more rapidly because coagulation factors become unstable after thawing. • Only one person must identify blood product and patient.	• Administer ABO group-specific or compatible. Rh type compatibility is generally not required because product doesn't contain RBCs. • Adverse reactions are usually slight, with febrile nonhemolytic and allergic urticarial reactions most common. • Administer within 6 hours of thawing because coagulation factors lose potency at room temperature. (Generally, unit can be safely transfused in 2 hours.)

continued

GUIDE TO BLOOD PRODUCTS *continued*

BLOOD PRODUCT	DESCRIPTION	INDICATIONS	EQUIPMENT
Platelet concentrates	30- to 60-ml unit contains about half of original platelets in unit of whole blood	• Thrombocytopenia • Thrombocytopathy	• Same as for whole blood, except: —use component Y set when administering *I.V. drip* so you can rinse pack with normal saline to ensure transfusion of all platelets; also, filter with smaller surface area is less likely to trap platelets. To administer *I.V. push,* use component syringe set. —all tubing should be rubber-free to prevent platelets from sticking to it.
Cryoprecipitated antihemophilic factor	Frozen 20-ml unit contains mostly coagulation factor VIII, plus 250 mg of fibrinogen	• Hemophilia A • Von Willebrand's disease • Hypofibrinogenemia • "Fibrin glue"	• Same as for whole blood, except: —smaller needle or catheter size (22G or 23G for adults) may be used because product is not viscous. —use component Y set if available (same rationale as for platelet concentrates). —product won't stick to rubber.
Granulocytes	Units vary in volume (200 to 500 ml), but contain mostly granulocytes (number depends on method of salvage), plus RBCs, plasma, and platelets.	• Severe gram-negative infection or severe neutropenia, unresponsive to routine therapy, in immunosuppressed patient • Severe granulocyte dysfunction	• Same as for whole blood, but microaggregate filter is contraindicated because it would trap granulocytes.
Serum albumin (5% and 25%) and plasma protein fraction (PPF)	25% albumin, which contains higher concentration of albumin than 5%, comes in 50-ml and 100-ml units. 5% albumin and PPF (essentially same product) come in 250-ml units.	• Hypovolemia • Hypoproteinemia (for example, in burn patients)	• Same as for whole blood, but because product comes in glass bottle, use administration set supplied with it, which will have filtered air inlet. Also, normal saline needn't be used as starter solution. Needs no blood filter.

ADMINISTRATION	SPECIAL CONSIDERATIONS
• Same as for whole blood, but transfuse more rapidly to prevent platelets from clumping and sticking to side of bag.	• Administer ABO group- and Rh type-compatible if possible. • Inspect unit for color. It should have yellow tinge. • Agitate bag more often than other blood products because platelets tend to clump. • Adverse reactions are usually slight. • American Red Cross recommends that units of platelet concentrates be pooled in blood bank into transfer packs, rather than administered as single-donor units. Expiration date is usually 2 to 5 days from date of collection, depending on method of storage. • One apheresis platelet unit collected from one donor equals 6 to 8 units of platelet concentrate.
• Same as for whole blood, but transfuse more rapidly because coagulation factors become unstable after thawing. • Only one person must identify blood product and patient. • Vital signs can be taken p.r.n.	• Administer ABO group-compatible. Rh type compatibility not required. • Patient usually receives multiple units. American Red Cross recommends that blood bank pool number of units ordered into transfer packs. Administer all units within 6 hours of thawing. • Watch for adverse reactions like those that most commonly follow plasma transfusions. • Because product has short half-life, transfusions may need to be repeated frequently, depending on patient's clinical status.
• Same as for whole blood, but transfuse slowly to aid patient tolerance.	• Administer ABO group-compatible and, when possible, Rh type- and human leukocyte antigen-compatible too. (For best results, administer as soon as possible after salvage.) • Lifesaving procedure that must be repeated daily for 4 to 5 days or longer to be effective. • Because product consists of white blood cells, watch for chills and fever. Other typical reactions include coughing and shortness of breath. Continue transfusion if possible. But if severe dyspnea develops, stop transfusion, keep vein open, and notify doctor.

• Unlike whole blood in several respects:
  –25% albumin usually not given at rate exceeding 1 ml/min because of danger of fluid overload.
  –PPF given at over 10 ml/min may produce hypotension.
  –Only one person must identify product and patient.
  –Vital signs can be taken as necessary.
	• Compatibility testing not required because albumin and PPF contain no RBCs or plasma antibodies.
	• 25% albumin is used for patients whose vascular volume is depleted but who have extravascular fluid accumulation.
	• Because 25% albumin rapidly mobilizes large volumes of fluid into circulation, watch for pulmonary edema and other signs or symptoms of fluid overload.
	• Product is stored at room temperature and has extremely long shelf life. Always check expiration date before administering.

How to use a Y set for blood administration

Blood administration sets come with both straight and multiple-lead tubing. A Y set is a multiple lead tubing. This type of administration set minimizes the risk of contamination, especially for transfusion of multiple units of blood. The Y set allows you to administer other blood products or volume expanders safely and easily; it also provides the option of adding normal saline solution to make the packed RBCs less viscous.

NOTE If the patient can't tolerate the extra fluid, don't add normal saline.

1 To use the Y set correctly, begin by examining the line shown here. Note that the filter is inside the drip chamber.

Now, move the roller clamp on the main line directly under the drip chamber, or as near to it as possible, and close it. Make sure you close the clamps on the saline solution line and the clamp on the blood line.

2 Remove the cap from the spike on the saline solution line. Insert the spike into the container.

3 Remove the cap from the blood line spike. Then, expose the blood bag's port by pulling back the two tabs at the top of the bag.

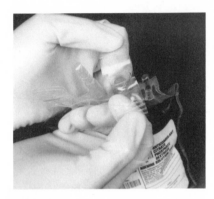

NOTE Don't touch the port or you'll contaminate it. Insert the blood line spike into the blood bag port.

4 Hang the entire Y set on an I.V. pole.

Change the Y set tubing every 4 hours, or according to institution policy.

5 While making sure the clamp on the blood line is closed, open the saline line clamp. Squeeze the combination drip chamber and filter until it's half full. Then open the main tubing clamp and flush the entire line with saline solution. Close both clamps.

To dilute the packed RBCs, position the blood lower than the saline. Keep both Y clamps open. Allow 50 to 75 ml of saline to backflow into the blood bag, then clamp the tubings. Gently rock the blood bag to distribute the normal saline.

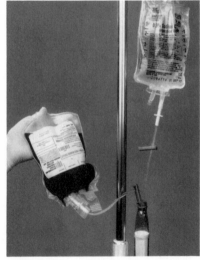

6 Remove the primary I.V. tubing. Attach a needle with a cap to protect the end of the primary tubing. Attach the blood tubing to the venipuncture device.

7 Open the saline solution clamp and the main flow rate clamp to flush the entire line with saline solution. Then, close both clamps.

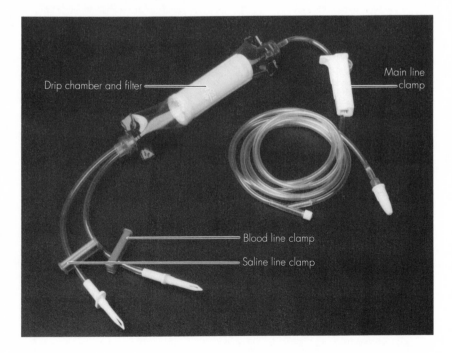

Drip chamber and filter

Main line clamp

Blood line clamp

Saline line clamp

GUIDE TO REQUESTING AND IDENTIFYING BLOOD PRODUCTS

Because blood is delicate and costly, all institutions have strict guidelines for obtaining blood. These guidelines may vary from one institution to another, so consult your procedure manual to learn the protocol for obtaining a blood product from your blood bank.

Remember that you can't return a unit of packed RBCs to a blood bank for reissue if it's been out of a monitored environment for more than 30 minutes, so request packed RBCs from the blood bank only when you're ready to administer them. A monitored environment is one in which the temperature stays between 33.8° and 42.8° F (1° and 6° C), the acceptable range for packed RBCs. Refrigerators equipped with an alarm that sounds when the temperature is outside that range provide such an environment. They're found in the blood bank itself and sometimes in an operating room suite.

Commonly, the worst adverse reactions to blood transfusions result from failure to correctly identify the blood product or the patient. After the blood product has been brought to the nursing unit, it must be identified to make sure it's the right one to transfuse. The patient must also be identified. At least two persons (in many institutions, two registered nurses) must perform this step. To identify the blood product:
• Check the compatibility tag attached to the blood bag and the information printed on the bag itself to verify that the ABO group, Rh type, and unit number match.
• For whole blood, check the patient's ABO group and his RH type, which should be on his chart and his identification bracelet, to confirm that they match those on the compatibility tag and blood bag. Do the same for group- and type-*specific* packed RBCs. For group- and type-*compatible* RBCs, compare the patient's ABO group and Rh type with the crossmatch results on the compatibility tag.
• Make sure the blood product matches the order on the patient's chart.
• Check the expiration date on the blood bag.
• Inspect the blood product for clots, and look for a purplish tinge or excessive bubbling, which may indicate bacterial contamination.

If you find any discrepancies between the information on the compatibility tag and blood bag and that on the patient's chart and identification bracelet, report them to the blood bank immediately and postpone the transfusion until the discrepancies have been corrected.

Blood type compatibility

Precise blood typing and cross matching are essential. If the donor's blood is incompatible with the recipient's, the transfusion can be fatal. In most instances, determining the recipient's blood type and cross matching it with available donor blood takes less than 1 hour.

The four blood groups are distinguished by their agglutinogen (antigen in RBCs) and their agglutinin (antibody in serum or plasma).

The following shows donor-recipient blood group compatibility:

Recipient	Donor
A	A, AB
B	B, AB
AB	AB
O	A, B, AB, O

8 Open the blood line clamp. Squeeze the combination drip chamber and filter on the Y set until the filter's completely immersed in blood.

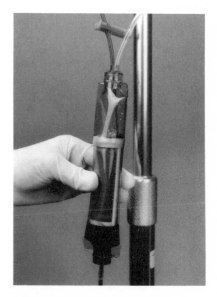

9 Open the Y set's main clamp, and adjust the blood's flow to the prescribed rate.

10 When the blood bag is empty, close the blood line clamp. Open the saline solution clamp to flush the tubing with saline solution. Then close the remaining clamps.

11 Remove the blood tubing and reattach the primary tubing. Readjust the I.V. flow rate. Document your actions.

How to use a leukocyte-removal filter

A patient who receives multiple blood transfusions may develop antibodies against certain blood components, particularly leukocytes. Patients who require repeated transfusions but who have developed HLA antibodies against transfused leukocyte antigens may receive transfusions of leukocyte-poor RBCs or leukocyte-poor whole blood. Any unit of blood can be made leukocyte poor by adding a leukocyte-removal filter to the blood bag.

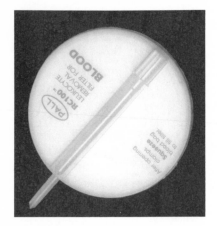

This filter removes about 99% of the leukocytes in the blood. The following photos describe how to use the Pall leukocyte-removal filter for blood transfusion.

1 Attach the spike of the blood administration set to the leukocyte-removal filter.

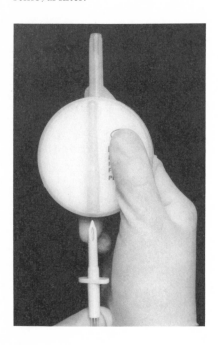

2 Attach the upper spike of the filter to the blood bag, as shown.

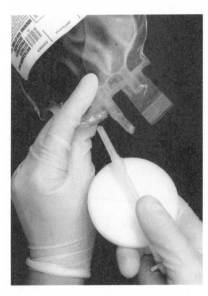

3 Open the clamp on the blood administration set. Gently squeeze the blood bag to prime the filter.

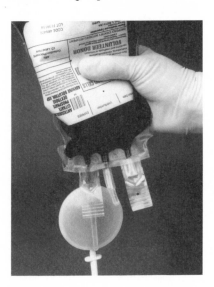

4 Prime the tubing and clamp it off. You are now ready to begin the blood transfusion.

NOTE During the transfusion, do not squeeze the drip chamber. This may cause air entrapment in the filter.

NURSING TIP When adding a second unit of blood, clamp the tubing to the leukocyte-removal filter. If air enters the filter it may reduce the rate of blood flow. A pressure cuff may also be used to hasten the transfusion (see How to use a Built-in Blood Pump).

How to use a built-in blood pump

If your patient needs large amounts of blood fast, use a blood pump. You have three types of pumps to choose from: a pump that's built into the Y set, like the one shown here, a pump that you slip onto the blood bag, or an electronic infusion pump.

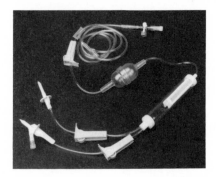

Before using an electronic infusion pump to deliver blood, check the manufacturer's recommendations.

The following photos show how to use the built-in pump, which operates with manual pressure.

1 Close the upper and lower flow clamps. Remove the spike cover.

2 Holding the blood bag securely, pull back the two tabs at the top to expose the port. Insert the spike with a twisting motion, making sure it's snug.

3 Squeeze the combination drip chamber and filter until it begins to fill. Continue squeezing it until the filter's completely immersed in blood. Tap the chamber to expel any trapped air bubbles.

4 Invert the lower pump chamber, as shown. Open both clamps.

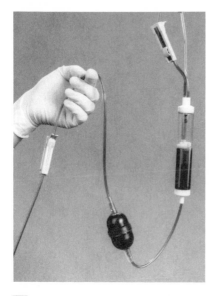

5 Holding the needle adapter upright, prime the tubing. Make sure you expel any trapped air bubbles.

Now, close the lower clamp. Then remove and cap the primary tubing with a needle. Connect the blood pump line to the venipuncture device. Avoid piggybacking blood tubing into a Y site on a primary I.V. set. Prime the primary line with normal saline solution (see How to Use a Y Set for Blood Administration, pages 168 and 169).

6 Now you're ready to administer the blood. Open both clamps all the way. Squeeze and release the pump chamber to force blood down the tubing.

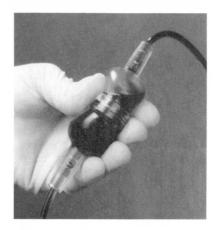

7 Be sure to let the pump chamber refill completely before squeezing and releasing it again. Continue doing this until the blood bag is empty.

NOTE If you want to stop using the pump before the blood bag is completely emptied, simply stop pumping and adjust the flow rate.

How to use a slip-on blood pump

Another type of pump you can use when you want to administer large amounts of blood quickly is the slip-on type, shown here.

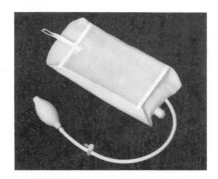

It slips right over the blood bag. To use it correctly, follow these instructions:

1 Insert the spike of the blood administration set into the blood bag and prime the tubing.

2 Insert your hand into the pump envelope, and pull the blood bag up through the center opening.

3 Grasp the pump envelope loops used for hanging and slip them through the blood bag loop. Then, hang the set on an I.V. pole as shown.

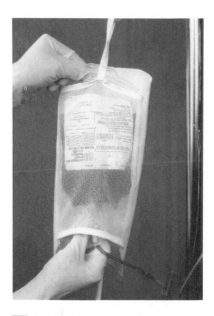

4 Turn the stopcock to the right, as in the off position shown.

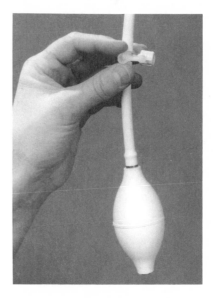

Next, connect the line to the venipuncture device and open the flow clamp on the administration set.

5 Squeeze the bulb of the pump until you've reached the desired flow rate.

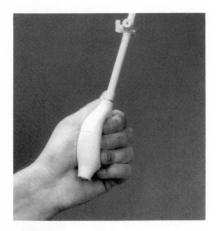

NOTE Don't let the pressure on the pump exceed 300 mm Hg. At that level, the pressure's so great it may damage the red blood cells, cause the line to disconnect, or rupture the bag.

6 Turn the stopcock to the off position to maintain a constant pressure rate.

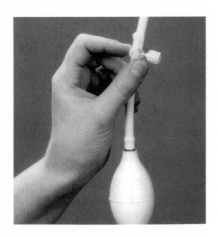

Repeat the procedure with each new blood bag. Remember, as the bag empties, pressure decreases. Check the flow rate and adjust the clamp, as necessary. Observe the site carefully. If the vein's too small to accept blood under pressure, the blood may infiltrate the skin.

TROUBLESHOOTING TRANSFUSION PROBLEMS

You can give your patient the best care possible during a transfusion and still encounter problems. But if you anticipate some of the more common difficulties and know how to deal with them, you can manage the situation well.

If the transfusion stops running:
• Check the distance between the I.V. container and the insertion site. Make sure it's at least 3' (90 cm) above the site.
• Check the flow clamp to make sure it's open.
• Observe the filter to see if it's completely immersed in blood.
• Rock the bag back and forth gently to agitate blood cells that may have settled to the bottom.
• Squeeze the tubing and flashbulb to get the fluid moving again.
• Untape the dressing over the insertion site, and make sure the needle or catheter's still correctly placed in the vein. Reposition it, if necessary.
• Close the main line flow clamp. Lower the blood bag and open the saline solution line. Dilute the blood with 50 to 100 ml of saline to facilitate blood flow.

If a hematoma's developing at the needle site:
• Stop the infusion immediately.
• Remove the needle or catheter, and cap the tubing with a new needle and guard.
• Notify the doctor. He'll probably want you to place ice on the site for 24 hours and warm compresses after that.
• Promote reabsorption of the hematoma by gently exercising the involved limb.
• Document your actions and observations.

If the blood bag's empty and the new unit hasn't arrived from the blood bank:
• Hang a container of normal saline solution (if you haven't already), and administer it slowly until the new unit arrives.
• If you're using a Y set, close the blood line clamp, open the saline solution line clamp, and let the saline solution run slowly until the new unit arrives. Make sure you decrease the flow rate or clamp the line before you attach the new unit of blood.

Learning about blood and fluid warmers

A blood or fluid warmer is a device that provides external heat to blood or intravenous fluid before it enters the patient's vein. This device may be electronic or nonelectronic. It may require special tubing, a warming bag, or it may be used with conventional blood administration sets. Before using any blood or fluid warmer, be sure to read the manufacturer's instructions. Also, check institution policy regarding the use of a blood or fluid warmer.

Blood or fluid warmers may be used to:
• prevent hypothermia and patient discomfort during rapid delivery of a large volume of cold blood
• prevent cardiac arrhythmia during central line blood administration
• prevent an antigen-antibody reaction when cold agglutinins are identified in the cross matching process; cold agglutinins may cause clumping at temperatures below 39° F (4° C), leading to hemolysis.

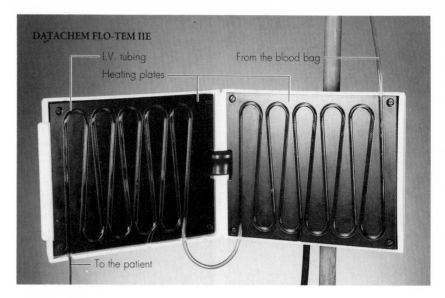

DATACHEM FLO-TEM IIE

I.V. tubing

Heating plates

From the blood bag

To the patient

How to use a Data Chem Flo-Tem IIe blood or fluid warmer

1 Prepare the blood bag and prime the tubing as discussed on pages 168 and 169. Use extra long blood administration tubing to extend the warming area (Flo-Tem warmers use standard I.V. or extension tubing).

2 Turn on the warmer. Next, open the door and insert the blood administration tubing into the recessed channels of the device.

3 Close the door and regulate the flow rate as usual. Document the use of this device in your nurse's notes.

NOTE   An alarm will sound if the temperature of the blood warmer exceeds 104° F (40° C).

Autotransfusion: A growing role in surgical care

Thanks to safer, simpler equipment and techniques, autotransfusion (the collection, filtration, and reinfusion of a patient's own blood) has become a widely accepted procedure in emergency departments and trauma centers. Used mostly for patients with chest wounds, it's indicated whenever 2 or 3 units of pooled blood can be recovered from a wound or body cavity.

Autotransfusion also plays an important part in nonemergency surgery. Blood may be obtained:
• *preoperatively.* A patient can donate his blood for storage and later use during elective surgery up to 35 days in advance. He can donate as often as every 5 days up to 5 days before surgery. Even patients with conditions that normally rule out blood donation can donate for autotransfusion.
• *immediately before surgery.* After anesthetizing the patient, the doctor can withdraw 1 to 2 units of blood and replace the volume with a crystalloid or colloid solution to provide fresh, warm, compatible blood for immediate use. This procedure is

most common in cardiovascular and orthopedic procedures.
• *during surgery.* The doctor can collect shed blood from a wound or body cavity, process it, and then reinfuse it.
• *postoperatively.* Blood shed during surgery can be collected and replaced in the recovery room, surgical intensive care unit, or orthopedic unit.

Pros and cons

The doctor may order autotransfusion instead of a stored blood transfusion because autotransfusion:
• eliminates the risk of transfusion reactions and transmission of such diseases as hepatitis, malaria, and acquired immunodeficiency syndrome
• provides compatible blood immediately by eliminating the usual 45-minute period required for blood typing and cross matching
• reduces transfusion costs (blood for autotransfusion is up to six times cheaper per unit than donor blood)
• prevents transfusion hypothermia because the blood's already warm
• avoids hypokalemia, hypocalcemia, and acidosis because the blood has normal levels of potassium, ammo-

TRANSFUSION RISKS: IMMEDIATE REACTIONS

Transfusion reactions can occur during, immediately after, or up to 96 hours after any blood transfusion. They're primarily caused by incompatibility, contaminated blood, or too rapid an infusion.

Study this chart to learn what to look for, how to treat the reactions, and how to prevent them from happening again.

REACTION	CAUSE	SIGNS AND SYMPTOMS	TREATMENT
Air embolism (uncommon but possibly fatal)	Air in bloodstream via tubing	Blood foaming in heart, with subsequent pumping inability, causing shock	Treat for shock. Turn patient on his left side, with his head down.
Allergic (common but not serious)	Atopic substance in blood	Pruritus, urticaria, facial swelling, chills, fever, nausea, vomiting	Notify doctor. Administer parenteral antihistamines or, for more serious cases, epinephrine (Adrenalin) or steroids, as ordered.
Blood contamination (uncommon but serious)	Presence of gram-negative *Pseudomonas*, coliform or achromobacteria	Chills, fever, hypotension, vomiting, diarrhea, shock	Treat with antibiotics and steroids, as ordered.
Circulatory overload (common and treatable)	Too large an infusion	Engorged neck veins; constricted chest with breathing difficulties; flushed feeling; moist rales; eventually, acute edema	Keep the primary line open with dextrose 5% in water (not saline solution). Notify doctor immediately for possible administration of diuretics, rotating tourniquets, or phlebotomy therapy.
Febrile (common but not serious)	Presence of bacterial lipopolysaccharides; recipient's anti-HLA antibodies react with transfused lymphocytes or platelet cell membranes	From mild chills, fever, to extreme symptoms resembling hemolytic reaction.	For mild cases, administer antipyretics and antihistamines as ordered. For severe cases, treat like hemolytic reaction
Hemolytic (uncommon but possibly fatal)	ABO or Rh incompatibility, or improper storage	Chills, fever, low back pain, chest pain, hypotension, nausea, vomiting, and bleeding abnormalities. Usually rapid onset after start of blood administration	Stop transfusion. Keep the vein open by connecting a secondary line of normal saline solution to the blood line. Correct shock by administering oxygen, fluids, and epinephrine as ordered. Maintain renal circulation by administering mannitol (Osmitrol) or furosemide (Lasix). Collect blood and urine samples for the laboratory. Blood will show hemolysis, and urine will contain hemoglobin. Carefully record fluid intake and output after discontinuation of blood. Watch for diuresis or oliguria.
Plasma protein incompatibility (uncommon but serious)	IgA incompatibility	Flushing, abdominal pain, diarrhea, chills, fever, dyspnea, hypotension	Treat for shock by administering oxygen, fluids, and epinephrine, as ordered. Sometimes steroids are administered.

PREVENTION

- Expel air from tubing before starting transfusion.
- Monitor the infusion.

- Determine if the patient reacted allergically to previous transfusions. If he did, he has a two-in-three chance of experiencing it again.

- Use air-free, touch-free methods to draw and deliver blood.
- Maintain strict storage control.
- Use aseptic technique when warming infusion.
- Change the filter and tubing every 4 hours, and the blood at least every 4 hours.

- Use packed RBCs instead of whole blood.
- Infuse at a reduced rate (by using an electronic control device, for example) for high-risk patients
- Keep the patient warm and in a sitting position.
- Use a diuretic when beginning the transfusion.

- Keep patient covered and warm.
- Use a leukocyte-removal filter during transfusion.
- Use saline-washed RBCs or frozen saline-washed packed cells.
- Administer antipyretic medications with the blood.
  Important: Never add antihistamines to the blood bag.

- Double-check the patient's identification and blood type to make sure blood is compatible.
- Begin transfusion slowly.
- Remain with patient for the first 20 minutes of the transfusion.

- Transfuse only IgA-deficient blood or well washed RBCs.

---

nia, hydrogen ions, and 2, 3-diphosphoglycerate, which helps oxygenate tissues
• reduces the risk of overtransfusion and subsequent circulatory overload
• conserves stored blood supplies
• may be given to patients with rare blood types and those with religious objections to homologous blood transfusions.

Possible complications of autotransfusion include hematologic changes (such as decreased platelet and fibrinogen levels and abnormal platelet function), coagulopathy, sepsis, microembolism, and air embolism.

How to use the Pleur-evac ATS
On the following pages, you'll learn how to use the Pleur-evac ATS. This autotransfusion device reduces the risk of error during an emergency and contains special equipment that minimizes blood cell damage during collection, reduces the risk of air embolism during transfusion, and filters out microaggregates.

1 Establish underwater seal drainage and connect the patient's chest tube by following the steps printed on the front of the Pleur-evac unit.

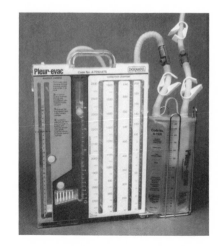

TRANSFUSION RISKS: TRANSMITTABLE DISEASES

You can never be sure the blood you're infusing is disease-free; no test will *always* identify transmittable diseases. This chart will help you identify some of the diseases that can be transmitted by transfusion, tell you how to treat them effectively, and how to prevent them from occurring in other patients.

DISEASE	CAUSE	INCUBATION TIME	CONFIRMATION
Acquired immunodeficiency syndrome (AIDS)	Presence of human immunodeficiency virus (HIV) in blood	Months to years; antibodies develop within 6 weeks to 6 months after infection. Presence of antibodies confirm presence of virus.	Enzyme-linked immunosorbent assay (ELISA) and the Western blot assay (two blood tests to detect HIV antibodies)
Hepatitis	Presence of hepatitis B and hepatitis C in blood (greatest risk in pooled plasma, fibrinogen, concentrates of factors VIII and IX; no risk in immune serum, globulin, plasma protein fraction (PPF), normal serum albumin) Hepatitis C (formerly called non-A, non-B) accounts for 85% of blood-borne hepatitis	2 weeks to 6 months	Make sure the blood is tested for hepatitis B and C antigens before administering it. Patient will have anorexia, vomiting, abdominal discomfort, enlarged liver, diarrhea, headache, fever, and jaundice.
Malaria	Presence of protozoan parasites within the RBCs	2 weeks to 4 months	Test blood for Plasmodium species.
Syphilis	Spirochetemia caused by *Treponema pallidum*	4 to 18 weeks	Check blood for syphilis with a serologic test, but don't consider results absolutely reliable. You can, however, consider a chancre positive proof of syphilis.
Viral syndrome	Presence of cytomegalovirus (CMV) or Epstein-Barr virus in the blood	2 to 5 weeks	The patient will show signs of fever; hepatitis to varying degrees, with or without jaundice; atypical lymphocytosis; rash.

TREATMENT	PREVENTION
Antiviral drugs reduce infectivity but do not cure HIV infection.	• Strict selection of donors; donor testing education; universal precautions. • Caregivers should observe blood and body fluid precautions.
Isolation, gamma globulin therapy, supportive treatment.	• Select reliable, healthy blood donors. • Conduct epidemiologic follow-ups of suspected cases to potential carriers. • Conduct radioimmunoassays for hepatitis B on all donor blood products. • Make sure blood is tested for the Australia antigen and the anti-hepatitis C virus.
Administer quinine sulfate (Legatrin) or chloroquine phosphate (Aralen Phosphate).	• Select only those donors who have not lived in endemic areas or have not taken anti-malarial drugs for at least 3 years.
Administer penicillin.	• Don't administer blood unless it's been tested and refrigerated for at least 2 days at 39.2° F (4° C) to kill spirochetes.
No specific therapy; let the reactions run their course.	• Select only those donors who are free from recent viral symptoms.

Inspect the blood collection bag and tubing, making sure all clamps are open and all connections airtight.

2 Add an anticoagulant, such as heparin or citrate phosphate dextrose, if prescribed, before collection. If citrate phosphate dextrose is prescribed, add one part to seven parts blood. Using an 18G (or smaller) needle, inject the anticoagulant through the red self-sealing port on the autotransfusion connector, as shown. The system's now ready to use. Chest cavity blood should begin collecting in the bag.

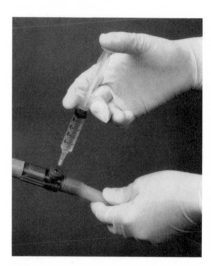

3 To collect more than one bag of blood, open a replacement bag when the first one's nearly full.

Close the clamps on top of the second bag. Before removing the first collection bag from the drainage unit, reduce excess negativity by using the high negativity relief valve. Depress the button, as shown; then release it when negativity drops to the desired level (watch the water seal manometer).

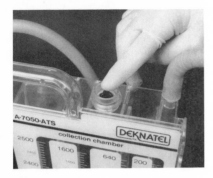

4 Close the white clamp on the patient tubing. Then, close the two white clamps on top of the collection bag.

5 Disconnect all connectors on the first bag. Attach the red (female) and blue (male) connector sections on top of the autotransfusion bag.

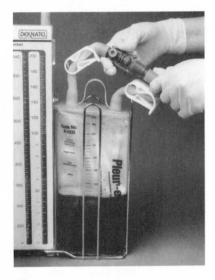

6 Remove the protective cap from the collection tubing on the replacement bag. Connect the collection tubing to the patient's chest drainage tube, using the red connectors.

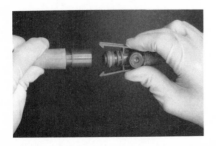

7 Remove the protective cap from the replacement bag's suction tube and attach the suction tube to the Pleur-evac unit, using the blue connectors. Make sure all connections are tight. Open all clamps and inspect the system for airtight connections.

8 Spread and disconnect the metal support arms, and remove the first bag from the drainage unit by disconnecting the foot hook.

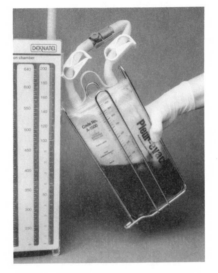

9 Use the foot hook and support arm to attach the replacement bag, as shown.

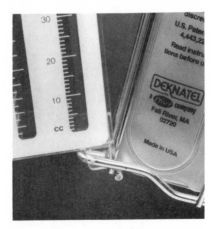

10 To reinfuse blood from the original collection bag, slide the bag off the support frame; then invert it so the spike port points upward.

NOTE Don't store collected blood; transfuse it within 6 hours of the start of collection.

11 Remove the protective cap from the spike port and insert a microaggregate filter into the port, using a twisting motion.

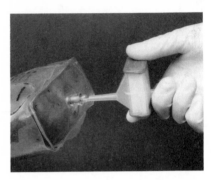

Prime the filter by gently squeezing the inverted bag. A new filter should be used with each bag.

12 Continue squeezing until the filter's saturated and the drip chamber's half full. Then, close the clamp on the reinfusion line and remove residual air from the bag. Invert the bag and suspend it from an I.V. pole; after carefully flushing the I.V. line to remove all air, infuse blood according to policy.

APPENDICES

A: Abbreviations Commonly Used in Drug Administration

ABBREVIATION	MEANING	ABBREVIATION	MEANING
a.c.	before meals	p̄	after
ad lib.	as often as desired	p.c.	after meals
b.i.d.	twice daily (while awake)	P.O. or p.o.	by mouth
g, G, or Gm	gram	P.R.N. or p.r.n.	as needed
gr	grain	pt	pint
gtt	drop	q.d.	every day
h or hr	hour	q.h.	every hour
h.s.	at bedtime	q.i.d.	four times daily (while awake)
I.M.	intramuscular	q2h, q3h, etc.	every 2 hours, every 3 hours, etc.
I.V.	intravenous	q.o.d.	every other day
kg	kilogram	q.s.	sufficient quantity
Ⓛ	left	Ⓡ	right
L or l	liter	s̄, s	without
mcg or μg	microgram	S.C., S.Q., or subq	subcutaneous
mEq	milliequivalent	SL or sl	sublingual
mg	milligram	s.o.s.	if needed
ml	milliliter	ss	one-half
mm	millimeter	stat	immediately
NPO	nothing by mouth	Tbs, or tbsp	tablespoon
od	every day	tsp or t	teaspoon
O.D.	right eye	t.i.d.	three times daily (while awake)
O.S.	left eye	U	unit
O.U.	both eyes	VO	verbal order
oz	ounce	w/ or c̄	with

B: Converting Units of Measure

This table provides approximate dose equivalents using the apothecary and metric systems of weights and measures. If the doctor prescribes a dosage form in the apothecary system, the pharmacist may supply a corresponding metric equivalent, and vice versa. Most medications are prepackaged and ready to administer, but it's useful to know what the equivalents are if you must calculate dosages yourself.

APOTHECARY EQUIVALENTS	METRIC EQUIVALENTS
Liquid measure	
1 quart	1,000 ml
1 1/2 pints	750 ml
1 pint	500 ml
8 fluidounces	250 ml
7 fluidounces	200 ml
3 1/2 fluidounces	100 ml
1 3/4 fluidounces	50 ml
1 fluidounce	30 ml
4 fluidrams	15 ml
2 1/2 fluidrams	10 ml
2 fluidrams	8 ml
1 1/4 fluidrams	5 ml
1 fluidram	4 ml
45 minims	3 ml
30 minims	2 ml
15 minims	1 ml
12 minims	0.75 ml
10 minims	0.6 ml
8 minims	0.5 ml
5 minims	0.3 ml
4 minims	0.25 ml
3 minims	0.2 ml
1 1/2 minims	0.1 ml
1 minim	0.06 ml
3/4 minim	0.05 ml
1/2 minim	0.03 ml

Converting weight

To begin, 1 lb equals 0.454 kg. Conversely, 1 kg equals 2.2 lb. To convert pounds to kilograms, divide the number of pounds by 2.2. To convert kilograms to pounds, multiply the number of kilograms by 2.2.

Converting temperature

To convert Celsius to Fahrenheit:

$$(°C \times 1.8) + 32 = °F$$

To convert Fahrenheit to Celsius:

$$(°F - 32) \div 1.8 = °C$$

Converting length

To begin, 1" equals 2.54 cm. Conversely, 1 cm equals 0.39". To convert inches to centimeters, divide the number of inches by 0.39. To convert centimeters to inches, multiply the number of centimeters by 0.39.

C: Calculating Dosages

Drug dosage calculations require a clear understanding of several mathematical concepts. You can gain this understanding by reviewing the concepts of ratios and proportions, by applying these concepts to various types of dose calculations, and by studying the step-by-step examples on the following pages.

Reviewing ratios and proportions

A *ratio* is a mathematical expression of the relationship between two different things. A *proportion* is a set of two equal ratios. A ratio may be expressed with a fraction, such as ⅓, or with a colon, such as 1:3.

When ratios are expressed as fractions in a proportion, their *cross products* are equal, as indicated below:

Proportion

$$\frac{2}{4} = \frac{5}{10}$$

Cross products

$$2 \times 10 = 4 \times 5$$

When ratios are expressed using colons in a proportion, the product of the means equals the product of the extremes:

Proportion

means

3 : 30 :: 4 : 40

extremes

Product of means and extremes

$$30 \times 4 = 3 \times 40$$

Whether fractions or ratios are used in a proportion, they must appear in the same order on both sides of the equal sign. When the ratios are expressed as fractions, the units in the numerators must be the same and the units in the denominators must be the same (although they do not have to be the same as the units in the numerators). The example below demonstrates this principle:

$$\frac{mg}{kg} = \frac{mg}{kg}$$

If the ratios in a proportion are expressed with colons, the units of the first term on the left side of the equal sign must be the same as the units of the first term on the right side. In other words, the units of the mean on one side of the equal sign must match the units of the extreme on the other side, and vice versa. The example below demonstrates this principle:

mg : kg :: mg : kg

Tips for simplifying dosage calculations

Leave units of measure in the calculation

This helps protect you from one of the most common dosage calculation errors—the incorrect unit of measure. When you leave units of measure in the calculation, those in the numerator and the denominator cancel each other out and leave the correct unit of measure in the answer. The following example uses the units of measure in calculating a drug with a usual dose of 4 mg/kg for a 55-kg patient:

• State the problem in a proportion:

   4 mg : 1 kg :: X mg : 55 kg

• Solve for X by applying the principle that the product of the means equals the product of the extremes:

   1 kg × X mg = 4 mg × 55 kg

• Divide and cancel out the units of measure that appear in the numerator and denominator:

$$X = \frac{4 \text{ mg} \times 55 \text{ kg}}{1 \text{ kg}}$$

X = 220 mg

Watch the zeros and decimal places

Suppose you receive an order to administer 0.1 mg of epinephrine S.C., but the only epinephrine on hand is a 1-ml ampule that contains 1 mg of epinephrine. To calculate the volume for injection, use the ratio and proportion method:

State the problem in a proportion:

   1 mg : 1 ml :: 0.1 mg : X ml

• Solve for X by applying the principle that the product of the means equals the product of the extremes:

   1 ml × 0.1 mg = 1 mg × X ml

• Divide and cancel out the units of measure that appear in the numerator and denominator, carefully checking the decimal placement:

$$\frac{1 \text{ ml} \times 0.1 \text{ mg}}{1 \text{ mg}} = X$$

$$0.1 \text{ ml} = X$$

Recheck calculations that seem unusual
For example, if a calculation yields an answer that suggests you administer 25 tablets, you've probably made a calculation error and should recheck your figures carefully. If you still have any doubt about your methods or results, review your calculations with another health care professional.

Determining the number of tablets to administer

Calculating the number of tablets to administer lends itself to the use of ratios and proportions. Follow this four-step process:

1. Set up the first ratio with the known tablet strength.
2. Set up the second ratio with the unknown quantity.
3. Use these ratios in a proportion.
4. Solve for X by applying the principle that the product of the means equals the product of the extremes.

For example, suppose a drug order calls for propranolol 100 mg P.O. q.i.d., but the only available form of propranolol is 40-mg tablets. You can use the four-step process to determine how many tablets to administer.

1. Set up the first ratio with the known tablet strength:

40 mg : 1 tab

2. Set up the second ratio with the desired dose and the unknown number of tablets:

100 mg : X tab

3. Use these ratios in a proportion:

40 mg : 1 tab :: 100 mg: X tab

4. Solve for X by applying the principle that the product of the means equals the product of the extremes:

$$1 \text{ tab} \times 100 \text{ mg} = 40 \text{ mg} \times X \text{ tab}$$

$$X = \frac{1 \text{ tab} \times 100 \text{ mg}}{40 \text{ mg}}$$

$$X = 2\frac{1}{2} \text{ tablets}$$

Determining the amount of liquid medication to administer

To calculate this amount, you can also use ratios and proportions. Follow the same four-step process used in determining the number of tablets to administer.

For example, a patient is to receive 750 mg of amoxicillin oral suspension. The label reads *Amoxicillin (Amoxicillin Trihydrate) 250 mg/5 ml. Bottle contains 100 ml.* How many milliliters of amoxicillin solution should the patient receive?

1. Set up the first ratio with the known liquid medication's strength:

250 mg : 5 ml

2. Set up the second ratio with the desired dose and the unknown quantity:

750 mg : X ml

3. Use these ratios in a proportion:

250 mg : 5 ml :: 750 mg : X ml

4. Solve for X by applying the principle that the product of the means equals the product of the extremes:

$$5 \text{ ml} \times 750 \text{ mg} = 250 \text{ mg} \times X \text{ ml}$$

$$X = \frac{5 \text{ ml} \times 750 \text{ mg}}{40 \text{ mg}}$$

$$X = 15 \text{ ml}$$

Administering drugs measured in units

Drugs such as epinephrine, heparin, insulin, and some antibiotics are measured in units. When calculating dosage for these drugs, follow the same guidelines used in the ratio and proportion method.

Remember: Always check the drug order against the drug available. Some drugs measured in units are available in various concentrations. Make sure that concentrations are part of the calculation process to prevent a serious dosage error. For example, a drug order calls for 0.2 mg epinephrine S.C. stat. The ampule is labeled 1 ml or 1:1,000 epinephrine. You need to calculate the correct volume of drug to inject.

1. Determine the strength of the solution based on its unlabeled ratio:

1 : 1,000 epinephrine = 1 g/1,000 ml

2. Set up a proportion with this information and the desired dose:

1 g : 1,000 ml :: 0.2 mg : X ml

Before you can perform this calculation, however, you must convert grams to milligrams by using the conversion

1 g = 1,000 mg

3. Restate the proportion with the converted units and solve for X:

1,000 mg : 1,000 ml :: 0.2 mg : X ml

1,000 ml × 0.2 mg = 1,000 mg × X ml

$$\frac{1,000 \text{ ml} \times 0.2 \text{ mg}}{1,000 \text{ mg}} = X$$

0.2 ml = X

D: Estimating Body-Surface Area in Children

Pediatric drug dosages should be calculated on the basis of body-surface area or body weight. If your pediatric patient is of average size, find his weight and corresponding surface area on the first scale to the left. Otherwise, use the nomogram to the right: Lay a straightedge on the correct height and weight points for your patient, and observe the point where it intersects on the surface area scale at center.
Note: Don't use drug dosages based on body-surface area in premature or full-term newborns. Instead, use body weight.

FOR CHILDREN OF NORMAL HEIGHT AND WEIGHT

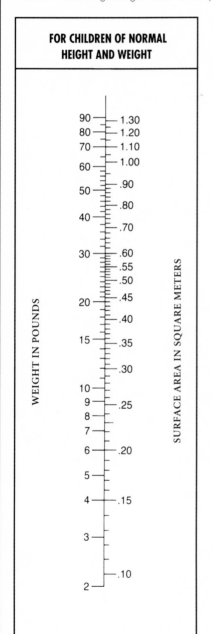

NOMOGRAM

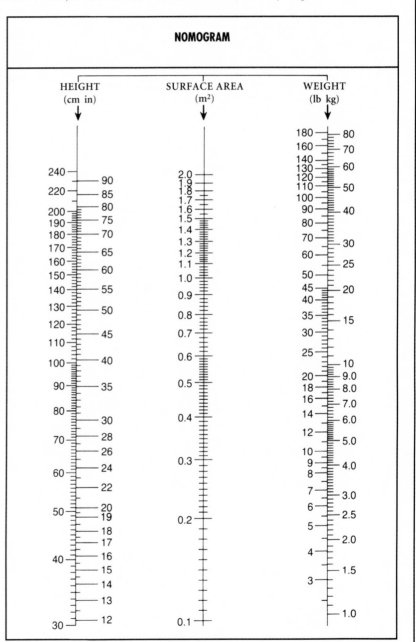

E: Estimating Body-Surface Area in Adults

Place a straightedge from the patient's height in the left-hand column to his weight in the right-hand column. The intersection of this line with the center scale reveals the body-surface area. The adult nomogram is especially useful in calculating dosages for chemotherapy.

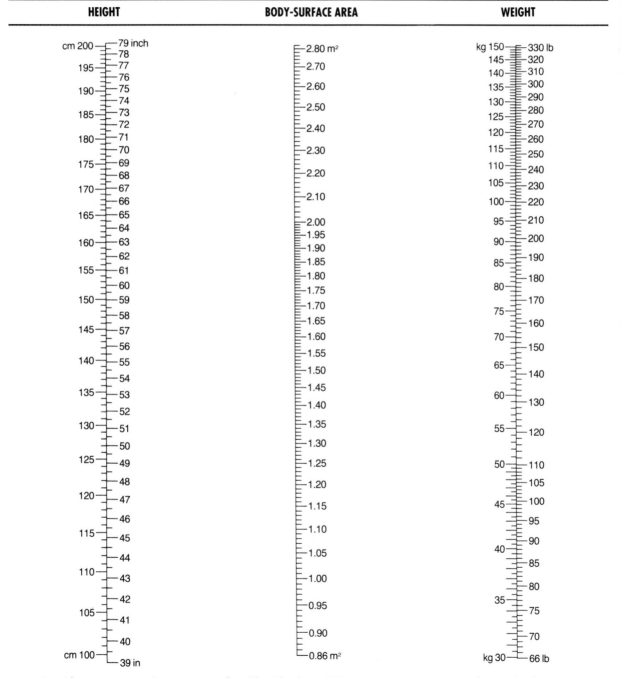

HEIGHT	BODY-SURFACE AREA	WEIGHT

Reproduced from Lentner, C. (ed.), *Geigy Scientific Tables*, 8th edition, 1986. Courtesy CIBA-GEIGY, Basel, Switzerland

F: I.V. Drug Compatibility

Use this chart only as a guide to drug compatibilities. Compatibility varies with the type, temperature, and volume of diluting solutions. Never combine two drugs if you're uncertain of their compatibility. Check appropriate references or with a pharmacist to be sure.

KEY:

- [shaded] , [8] = Compatible (Numbers indicate compatible only for hours indicated)
- [black] = Incompatible
- [white] = Data unavailable
- [diagonal] = Identical drug

	albumin	amikacin	aminophylline	amino acid injection	ampicillin	bretylium	calcium gluconate	carbenicillin	cefamandole	cefazolin	cefoxitin	cephalothin	chloramphenicol	cimetidine	clindamycin	corticotropin (ACTH)	dexamethasone	dextrose 5% in water	dextrose 5% in RL	dextrose 5% in 0.45% NSS	dextrose 5% in 0.9% NSS	diphenhydramine	dobutamine	dopamine	epinephrine	erythromycin lactobionate (I.V.)	gentamicin	heparin sodium	hydrocortisone Na succinate	insulin (regular)
albumin																														
amikacin			8				24	8		8			24	24	24		4	24	24	24	24	24		24					24	
aminophylline	8			24	48									24	24			24	24			24		24		24			24	
amino acid injection		24					24	24		24		24	24	24										24		24	24	24		24
ampicillin													1	24				2	4	4									6	
bretylium			48					48										48	48	48	48		48							48
calcium gluconate	24		24		48									24				24	24					24					24	
carbenicillin	8		24									24		24	24			24	24		24			24					24	
cefamandole																		24		48										
cefazolin	8		24									24	24	24				24												
cefoxitin														24				24	24	24	24						24			
cephalothin			24										24	24				24	24	24	24		6					24	24	
chloramphenicol	24			1					24					24				24	24		24									
cimetidine	24		24	24				24		24	24		24		24		24	24								24	24	24	48	24
clindamycin	24		24				24				24			24				24		24	24						24	24	24	
corticotropin (ACTH)																														
dexamethasone	4	24												24															4	4
dextrose 5% in water	24	24		2	48	24	24	24	24	24	24	24	24	24	24							48	24	24	6	24			24	
dextrose 5% in RL	24			4	48	24	24			24	24	24										48	48	24			24	24		
dextrose 5% in 0.45% NSS	24			4	48				48		24			24								48	48				24			
dextrose 5% in 0.9% NSS	24	24			48	24	24			24	24	24										48	48	24	6			24		
diphenhydramine	24																							24						
dobutamine																		48	48	48	48			24	24					
dopamine			24		48		24				6	24						24	48	48	48	24			24	24			24	18
epinephrine	24												24					24	24		24	24	24							
erythromycin lactobionate (I.V.)		24	24											24				6			6	24								
gentamicin			24							24			24	24				24			24									
heparin sodium			24							24		24		48	24		4	24	24				24							
hydrocortisone Na succinate	24	24		6			24				24			24			4	24	24				18							8
insulin (regular)			24		48									24				24										8		
isoproterenol			24															24	24		24								24	
kanamycin							48							24				24		24			24							
lactated Ringer's				8									24					48	48	24	18				24					
lidocaine	24	24		24	24								24					24		24	24	24	2		24		24			24
metaraminol	24		24										24					24	24	24	24									
methicillin			24										24					6	24	24	24					24				
methylprednisolone			24									24	24					6					18				24	4		
mezlocillin																		24												
moxalactam																		24	24	24	24									
multiple vitamin infusion								24						24				24	24		24									
nafcillin		24										48						24	24	24	24									
netilmicin																														
norepinephrine	24		24										24					24					24							
0.9% NSS	24	24		24	48	24	24	24	24	24	24	24	24	24	24							24	48	24	24	24	6	24		
oxacillin	8		24															6			12		24							
oxytocin																		6												
penicillin G potassium	8		24								24		24	24				24	24		24	24						24		
phytonadione	24		24										24						24										24	
piperacillin														24				24		24						24				
polymyxin B sulfate	24			1		1						24					24													
potassium chloride	4		24				24					24	24		4	24	24		24				24				24			
procainamide					24																24									
sodium bicarbonate	24	24		24	48		24			24	24			24				24		24					24		24	24	24	
tetracycline	4		24									24						24	24		24			24						
thiamine																		24												
ticarcillin			24															24												
tobramycin								24										24			48									
vancomycin	24													24				24												
verapamil		24	48		24	48	48	24	24	24	24	24	24	24	24			24	24		24		24		24	24	24	24	24	48
vitamin B complex with C													24					48	24		4	24								

Compatibility chart (columns left→right): isoproterenol, kanamycin, lactated Ringer's, lidocaine, metaraminol, methicillin, methylprednisolone, mezlocillin, moxalactam, multiple vitamin infusion, nafcillin, netilmicin, norepinephrine, 0.9% NSS, oxacillin, oxytocin, penicillin G potassium, phytonadione, piperacillin, polymyxin B sulfate, potassium chloride, procainamide, sodium bicarbonate, tetracycline, thiamine, ticarcillin, tobramycin, vancomycin, verapamil, vitamin B complex with C

Drug (row)	isoprot.	kanam.	lact.Ringer's	lidoc.	metaram.	methic.	methylpred.	mezloc.	moxal.	mult.vit.	nafcill.	netilm.	norepi.	0.9% NSS	oxacill.	oxytoc.	pen G K	phytonad.	piperac.	polymyxinB	KCl	procain.	Na bicarb	tetracyc.	thiam.	ticarc.	tobram.	vancom.	verap.	vit B w/C
albumin			24								24	24		8		8	24		24		4		24	4				24	24	
amikacin				24								24		24									24						48	
aminophylline	24		24	24	24	24								24	24		24	24		24			24							
amino acid injection			8											24					1		24							24		
ampicillin			24											48						24	48		48						48	
bretylium			24											24															48	
calcium gluconate														24					1	24	24								24	
carbenicillin														24															24	
cefamandole														24															24	
cefazolin		48								24				24							24					24	24		24	
cefoxitin														24							24								24	
cephalothin														24															24	
chloramphenicol	24		24	24		24				48	24	24			24	24	24	24		24			24			24	24		48	
cimetidine	24	24			24			24			24				24					24	24						24	24	
clindamycin																							4						
corticotropin (ACTH)																													4
dexamethasone	24	24		24	6	6	24	24	24	24			6	6	24		24	24	24		24	24			24	24		24	24
dextrose 5% in water	24		24	24	24		24	24	24			24		24				24	24		24								24
dextrose 5% in RL				24			24			24																			24
dextrose 5% in 0.9% NSS	24		24	24		24	24	24			12		24		24				24					48			24
diphenhydramine												24															24
dobutamine	24		48	24	24			24	24									24						24
dopamine	24	48	24		18			48	24									24	24				24
epinephrine	24	2					24														24
erythromycin lactobionate (I.V.)	18							24					24								24
gentamicin			24			24					24										24
heparin sodium	24		24		24				6	24			24				24				24
hydrocortisone Na succinate		24			4				24			24					24				24
insulin (regular)		24							24												48
isoproterenol		24							24												24
kanamycin		24							24												24
lactated Ringer's	24	24		24		24		24	24	24			24	24	24		24		24	24	48	24	24	24
lidocaine	24							24				24	24								48
metaraminol	24							24				24	24								24
methicillin	24							6				24								24
methylprednisolone								24												24
mezlocillin								6												
moxalactam	24							24												
multiple vitamin infusion	24				24		24	4			24	24								
nafcillin	24							24				24								
netilmicin				24																	
norepinephrine								24												24
0.9% NSS	24	24		24	24	6		6	24	24	24		8	24	24	24	24	24	24	48	24
oxacillin	24							8									24				24
oxytocin	24							24									24				24
penicillin G potassium	24				24		4	24									24				24
phytonadione	24																24				
piperacillin	24							24						24							
polymyxin B sulfate																					
potassium chloride	24						24	24			24		24				24				24
procainamide	24							24									24				
sodium bicarbonate	24	24				24		24	24	24	24		24				24				24
tetracycline	24					24		24								24					
thiamine	48							24													24
ticarcillin	24							48													24
tobramycin																					24
vancomycin	24		24	48	24	24	24				24	24	24	24	24			24		24	24	24	24		24
verapamil			24																		24

G: Calculating I.V. Infusion Rates

Calculating infusion rates for large-volume parenterals

For patients receiving large-volume parenterals (fluids given to maintain hydration or to replace fluids or electrolytes), you may have to convert the infusion rate to the volume administered over a period of time, such as 1 hour, 8 hours, or 24 hours. How you perform the calculations depends on how the original orders were written and how the institution requires orders to be written for large-volume parenterals. The calculations will vary, depending on whether you need to know the drip rate, the volume per hour, or the volume per shift or day.

To convert the infusion rate over a period of time, use this formula:

$$\frac{\text{Volume of fluid}}{\text{time in hours}} = \frac{\text{X ml}}{\text{1 hour}}$$

To calculate the drip rate, see below:

$$\frac{\text{Total number of ml}}{\text{total number of minutes}} \times \text{drip factor} = \text{drip rate}$$

HOW TO CALCULATE THE DRIP RATE: AN EXAMPLE

A doctor's order states: 500 ml of $D_5O.45NS$ to infuse over 12 hours. You need to determine the drip rate for an administration set that delivers 15 gtt/ml.

- Use the drip-rate equation:

$$\frac{\text{500 ml}}{\text{12 hr}} \times 60 \text{ min} \times 15 \text{ gtt/ml} = \text{X gtt/min}$$

- Multiply the number of hours by 60 minutes in the denominator of the fraction:

$$\frac{\text{500 ml}}{\text{720 min}} \times 15 \text{ gtt/ml} = \text{X gtt/min}$$

- Divide the fraction and solve for X:

$$0.69 \text{ ml/min} \times 15 \text{ gtt/ml} = \text{X gtt/min}$$
$$10.35 = \text{X gtt/min}$$

- Round the answer:

  10 gtt/minute

Calculating infusion rates when administering I.V. drugs

1 Determine the drug concentration in the infusion fluid.

2 Determine the dose to be administered per unit of time.

DRIP FACTORS

The drip factor is determined by the manufacturer of the equipment used when giving an I.V. infusion. Here are the drip factors of the various manufacturers.

MANUFACTURER	DROPS/MILLILITER
Abbott	15
Baxter Healthcare	10
Cutter	20
IVAC	20
McGaw	15

3 Identify the drip factor of the administration set to be used.

4 Convert all amounts to the same units of measure, such as all times to minutes, all volumes to milliliters, and all weights to milligrams.

5 If an infusion rate is ordered in mg/kg or mcg/kg, find the dose in milligrams or micrograms by multiplying the ordered dose by the patient's weight in kilograms.

When you have completed these steps, you can calculate the infusion rate by using this equation.

$$\text{Drug dose} \times \frac{1}{\text{drug concentration}} \times \text{drip factor} = \frac{\text{infusion}}{\text{rate}}$$

HOW TO USE THE INFUSION RATE EQUATION: TWO EXAMPLES

1. A doctor's order states: Add 2 g of lidocaine to 500 ml of D_5W and infuse at 2 mg/min. The microdrip set to be used will deliver 60 mcgtt/ml. You need to determine the infusion rate.

• State the drug dose: 2 mg/min

• State the drug concentration, converting it to like units and reducing it to its lowest terms, then inverting it to use the reciprocal (R) in the equation:

$$\frac{2\ g}{500\ ml} = \frac{2,000\ mg}{500\ ml} = \frac{4\ mg}{1\ ml} \ or \ \frac{1\ ml}{4\ mg} \ (R)$$

• Determine the drip factor: 60 mcgtt/ml

• Use these numbers in the infusion rate equation:

$$\frac{Drug}{dose} \times \frac{1}{concentration} \times \frac{drip}{factor} = \frac{infusion}{rate}$$

2 mg/min $\times$ 1 ml/4 mg $\times$ 60 mcgtt/1 ml = X

• Solve for X:

$$\frac{2\ mg}{1\ min} \times \frac{1\ mg}{4\ mg} \times \frac{60\ mcgtt}{1\ ml} = X$$

$$\frac{30\ mcgtt}{1\ min} = X$$

2. A doctor's order states: Add 50 mg of nitroprusside to 500 ml of D_5W and infuse at 2 mcg/kg/min. The patient weighs 60 kg. The microdrip set to be used will deliver 60 mgtt/ml. You need to determine the infusion rate.

• Determine the drug dose:
2mcg/kg/minute $\times$ 60 kg = 120 mcg/minute

• State the drug concentration, converting it to like units reduced to their lowest terms and inverted to give the reciprical for use in the equation:

$$\frac{50\ mg}{500\ ml} = \frac{1\ mg}{10\ ml} = \frac{1,000\ mcg}{10\ ml} = \frac{100\ mcg}{1\ ml}$$

or $\frac{1\ ml}{100\ mcg}$ (R)

• Determine the drip factor:

   60 mcgtt/ml

• Solve for X:

$$\frac{120\ mcg}{1\ min} \times \frac{1\ ml}{100\ mcg} \times \frac{60\ mcgtt}{1\ ml} = X$$

$$\frac{7,200\ mcgtt}{100\ min} = X$$

$$\frac{72\ mcgtt}{1\ min} = X$$

   60 mcgtt/ml = X

• Use these numbers in the infusion rate equation:

$$\frac{Drug}{dose} \times \frac{1}{concentration} \times \frac{Drip}{factor} = \frac{infusion}{rate}$$

$$\frac{120\ mcg}{1\ min} \times \frac{1\ ml}{100\ mcg} \times \frac{60\ mcgtt}{1\ ml} = X$$

You must express the drug concentration—usually written as g, mg, mcg/ml—in reciprocal (inverted) form. This places the milliliters in the numerator and the grams, milligrams, or micrograms in the denominator and allows the units of measure to cancel out appropriately. Adding units to the equation may clarify this step. If the drug dose appears in mg/minute, the drug concentration in mg/ml with the reciprocal ml/mg, and the drip factor in gtt/ml, the equation is:

mg/minute $\times$ ml/mg $\times$ gtt/ml = gtt/minute

GUIDE TO I.V. DRIP RATES

Use only if the infusion volume falls within the stated limits.

MANUFACTURER	DROPS/MINUTE TO INFUSE					
	100 ml/24 hr 21 ml/hr	51,000 ml/24 hr 42 ml/hr	1,000 ml/20 hr 50 ml/hr	1,000 ml/10 hr 100 ml/hr	1,000 ml/8 hr 125 ml/hr	1,000 ml/6 hr 166 ml/hr
Abbott	5	10	12	25	31	42
Baxter Healthcare	3	7	8	17	21	28
Cutter	7	14	17	34	42	56
IVAC	7	14	17	34	42	56
McGaw	5	10	12	25	31	42

Selected References

Bigelow-Kemp, B., Pillitteri, A., and Brown, P. *Fundamentals of Nursing,* 2nd ed. Glenview, Ill.: Scott, Foresman Co., 1989.

Clayton, B., and Stock, Y. *Basic Pharmacology for Nurses,* 9th ed. St. Louis: C.V. Mosby Co., 1989.

Cornwell, C.M. "The Ommaya Reservoir: Implications for Pediatric Oncology," *Pediatric Nursing* 16(3):249-257, May-June 1990.

Davis, N., and Cohen, M. "Learning from Mistakes: Medication Errors to Avoid," *Nursing87* 17(5):84-88, May 1987.

"Drugs and the Elderly: Basics Revisited 1987," *Geriatric Nursing* 8(5):270, September-October 1987.

Earnest, V. *Clinical Skills and Assessment Techniques in Nursing Practice.* Glenview, Ill.: Scott, Foresman Co., 1989.

Fiser, D.H. "Intraosseous Infusion," *New England Journal of Medicine* 322(22):1579-1581, May 31, 1990.

Hadaway, L.C. "A Midline Alternative to Central and Peripheral Venous Access," *Caring* 9(5):46-50, May 1990.

Hufler, D.R. "Helping Your Dysphagic Patient Eat," *RN* 50(9):36-38, 74, September 1987.

Kedzior, S. "Post-Spinal Anesthesia Headache and the Epidural Blood Patch," *Journal of Post Anesthesia Nursing* 1(4):258-259, November 1986.

Keen, M.F. "Get on the Right Track with Z-Track Injections," *Nursing90* 20(8):59, August 1990.

Jeglum, E. "Ocular Therapeutics," *Nursing Clinics of North America.*16(3):453-477, September 1981.

Illustrated Manual of Nursing Practice. Springhouse, Pa.: Springhouse Corp., 1991.

I.V. Therapy. Clinical Skillbuilders. Springhouse, Pa.: Springhouse Corp. 1990.

King, E., Wieck, L., and Dyer, M. *Illustrated Manual of Nursing Techniques,* 3rd ed. Philadelphia: J.B. Lippincott Co., 1986.

Lorenz, B. "Are You Using the Right I.V. Pump?" *RN* 53(5):31-37, May 1990.

Masoorli, S., and Angeles, T. "PICC Lines: The Latest Home Care Challenge," *RN* 53(1):44-51, January 1990.

McGovern, K. "10 Steps for Preventing Medication Errors," *Nursing86* 16(12):36-39, December 1986.

Medication Administration and I.V. Therapy Manual: Process and Procedures. Springhouse, Pa.: Springhouse Corp., 1988.

Metheny, N., Eisenberg, P., and McSweeney, H. "Effect of Feeding Tube Properties and Three Irrigants on Clogging Rates," *Nursing Research* 37(3)165-169, May-June 1988.

Millam, D.A. "Controlling the Flow: Electronic Infusion Devices," *Nursing90* 20(8):65-68, August 1990.

Morris, L.L. "Critical Care's Most Versatile Tool...A Multilumen Central Venous Catheter," *RN* 51(5):42-46, May 1988.

Nursing Photobook Annual. Springhouse, Pa.: Springhouse Corp., 1987.

Procedures. Nurse's Reference Library. Springhouse, Pa.: Springhouse Corp., 1985.

Rombeau, J., and Caldwell, M. *Atlas of Nutritional Support Techniques.* Boston: Little, Brown & Co., 1989.

Steele, J. *Practical I.V. Therapy.* Springhouse, Pa.: Springhouse Corp., 1988.

Timby, B.K. *Clinical Nursing Procedures.* Philadelphia: J.B. Lippincott Co., 1989.

Viall, C. "Your Complete Guide to Central Venous Catheters," *Nursing90* 20(2):34-42, February 1990.

Index

i refers to an illustration; t refers to a table.

i refers to an illustration; t refers to a table.

i refers to an illustration; t refers to a table.